EFT for SPORTS PERFORMANCE

Featuring Reports from EFT Practitioners,
Instructors, Students, and Users

by Gary Craig
www.EFTUniverse.com

Energy Psychology Press
P.O. Box 442, Fulton, CA 95439
www.energypsychologypress.com

Cataloging-in-Publication Data

Craig, Gary, 1940–

EFT for sports performance / by Gary Craig ; featuring reports
from EFT practitioners, instructors, students, and users. — 1st ed.

p. cm.

Includes index.

ISBN 978-1-60415-052-0

1. Emotional Freedom Techniques. 2. Sports—Physiological
aspects. 3. Athletes—training of. I. Title.

RC489.E45C73 2010

616.89'1—dc22

2010023395

© 2010 Gary Craig, www.EFTUniverse.com

Cover design by Victoria Valentine
Editing by CJ Puotinen
Typesetting by Karin Kinsey
Typeset in Cochin and Adobe Garamond
Printed in USA by Bang Printing
First Edition

10 9 8 7 6 5 4 3 2 1

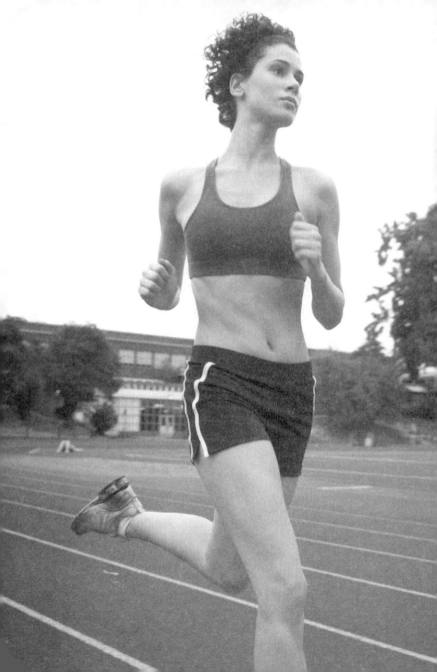

A Vital Guide for
Reading This Book

In a nutshell, EFT is an emotional version of acupuncture, except we don't use needles. Instead, we stimulate the acupuncture meridians by tapping on them with our fingertips. This often brings forth astonishing results that are likely beyond your expectations. The procedure is easy to learn and easy to use. You will learn the basics and more in this book.

EFT is good for everything. While this book focuses on EFT's use for improved sports performance, I must emphasize that **sports represent but a tiny fraction of EFT's long list of successes.** For example, EFT is good for pain and symptoms of all kinds and often works where nothing else will. It is also astonishingly useful for emotional issues of every type and reduces the typical psychotherapy process from months or years down to minutes or hours. Further, those wishing to improve their performance in school, business, public speaking, or the bedroom will also find EFT a valuable aid.

This book is like an encyclopedia. It is so comprehensive that it could easily be considered an "EFT

Encyclopedia for Improved Sports Performance." Most readers will not need to read it all, but every reader will want to keep it around as a priceless resource because it contains approaches and concepts that you will not find in other health-related books.

This book contains creative approaches written by many EFT experts. EFT is an "open source" healing tool that encourages experimentation. This means that we start with an easy-to-learn, simple procedure that works beautifully in the majority of cases. After that, anyone can experiment with the process and develop other refinements. Thus, for your expanded education, I am sprinkling within this book the opinions, refinements, and creative approaches of dozens of EFT'ers.

Depending on your interest level, previous experience, and individual response to EFT, there are several ways to read this book.

If you are new to EFT, I hope you may wish to start at the beginning and read it all the way through. By the time you reach the end, you will have an excellent chance of being completely and permanently free from sports performance problems in addition to having a thorough understanding of EFT and the ability to share this useful technique with friends and family.

If you're interested in the background of EFT and some of the technical, scientific, or engineering explanations that I'm fond of sharing, download our free EFT starter pack from the official EFT website, www.EFTUniverse.com. This book was designed as a companion to *The EFT Manual* and you'll learn something valuable from both.

For convenience, a condensed version of the manual is also available as a paperback book sold in retail bookstores and online. Look for *The EFT Manual (EFT: Emotional Freedom Techniques)* by Gary Craig, published by Energy Psychology Press, 2008.

If you're an experienced EFT'er, peruse the Table of Contents and go where your curiosity and interest take you. One of my goals in writing this book is to provide as many interesting examples as possible, so that all of us —including EFT instructors and practitioners—can add to our repertoire of approaches and strategies for making EFT more effective and versatile.

Our books and trainings are vital to your complete comprehension of EFT. I would like to emphasize that this book and *The EFT Manual* do not contain everything there is to know about EFT. You can learn the basics, and then tap along with the EFT sessions you'll find at www.EFTUniverse.com, or at workshops and events, and you'll find your knowledge of EFT expanding dramatically. While tapping, you can collapse or neutralize issues that have until now interfered with your performance goals. See my description of Easy EFT in Appendix B for the fastest, simplest way to use EFT by combining video with tapping. There is more human drama, inspiration, and humor in our videotaped presentations than there is in any reality television show!

Our books and training sessions are also the foundation for professional certification. Whether you are already in the healing field, or interested in building an EFT practice, EFT instruction is the place to begin. Each level of EFT training has a corresponding Study Guide. Once you have completed your process with the Study Guide, you can obtain EFT Certification by meeting the requirements stated in the guide. Serious students are encouraged to use the Study Guides even if Certification is not a goal.

Contents

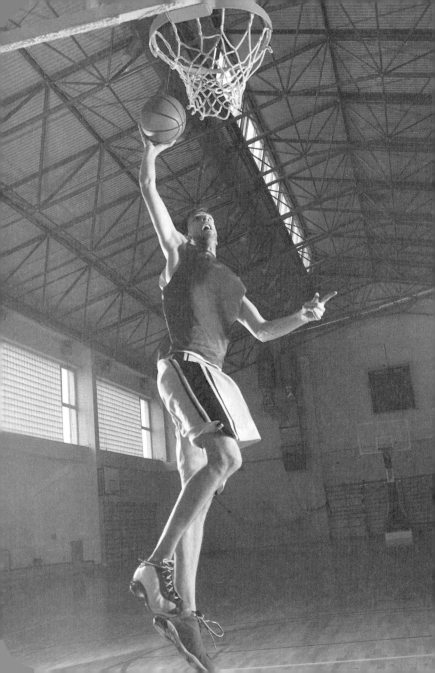

Notes and Acknowledgments

The list of individuals who contributed to the development of EFT can never be complete because most of them lived over 5,000 years ago. Those are the brilliant physicians who discovered and mapped the centerpiece of EFT, namely, the subtle energies that course through our bodies. These subtle energies are also the centerpiece of acupuncture and, as a result, EFT and acupuncture are cousins. Both disciplines are growing rapidly here in the West and, as time unfolds, they are destined to have a primary role in emotional and physical healing.

In the 20th Century, other dedicated souls advanced our use of ancient techniques that utilize the body's energy. Principal among them is Dr. George Goodheart, who developed Applied Kinesiology, a forerunner of EFT. In the 1960s, Dr. Goodheart discovered that muscle testing could be used to gather important information from the body, and he went on to train many health care practitioners and publish important books and papers.

Dr. John Diamond's work deserves applause because, to my knowledge, he was one of the first psychiatrists to use and write about these subtle energies. His many pioneering concepts, together with advanced ideas from Applied Kinesiology, have formed the foundation upon which our work is constructed. Dr. Diamond's best-sellers include *Life Energy: Using the Meridians to Unlock the Power of Your Emotions* (Continuum International, 1990) and *Life Energy and the Emotions* (Eden Grove, 1997).

Dr. Roger Callahan, the clinical psychologist from whom I received my original introduction to "emotional acupressure," deserves all the credit history can give him. He was the first to bring these techniques to the public in a substantial way and he did so despite open hostility from his own profession. As you might appreciate, it takes heavy doses of conviction to plow through the ingrained beliefs of conventional thinking. Without Roger Callahan's missionary drive, we might still be sitting around theorizing about this "interesting thing."

It is upon the shoulders of these giants that I humbly stand. My own contribution to the rapidly expanding field of meridian therapies has been to reduce the unnecessary complexity that inevitably finds its way into new discoveries. EFT is an elegantly simple version of these procedures, which professionals and laypeople alike can use on a variety of problems.

I also owe a special debt of gratitude to Adrienne Fowlie, who, through a friend, introduced me to meridian tapping techniques and helped me develop EFT.

Many EFT students and practitioners helped make this book possible. I am grateful to all who contributed case studies and reports. Most of the examples given here were published in our email newsletter and are posted in the newsletter's archives at the EFT website, www.EFTUniverse.com. The growth of this collection of reports has been something to behold. Awesome is an appropriate word, as there are so many articles in this collection that they could be bound into personalized reference books on many topics. Our website is loaded with some of the best of these contributions.

The names given in the reports presented here have often been changed to protect the privacy of those involved. This is especially likely if only first names are given. When a person's full name is given, it has not been changed and is used with permission.

In the interests of editorial consistency, reports from the United Kingdom, Australia, Canada, and other countries that use British spelling and punctuation have been changed to conform to standard American English.

Like most topics of special interest, EFT has its own language, words, or abbreviations that have special meaning for its students and practitioners. You'll find a list of EFT terms and their definitions in the Glossary.

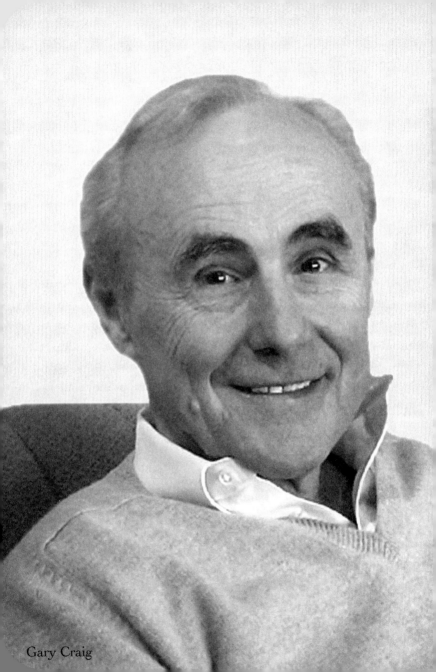
Gary Craig

Introduction

Two subjects that are most near and dear to my heart are EFT and sports. I've played just about every sport at least once, and in high school my main events were football, baseball, and basketball. I was offered football scholarships to 22 universities, which is how I attended Stanford University in California, and as a high school baseball player I was scouted by the Cleveland Indians. I never became a professional athlete, and these days I mostly run on the beach, but sports remain a major interest.

I've always appreciated the strong connection between emotions and performance. Athletes use terms like "being in the zone" to describe the effortless way in which they perform at their best, a state in which events seem to take place in slow motion and the athletes are completely relaxed, yet alert and focused. Then there's the opposite state in which the brain freezes, coordination departs, and nothing goes right.

Negative or doubting self-talk can leave one feeling defeated even before the game or event begins. Yet even though sports psychologists have made everyone aware of the mind/body connection, understanding the theory behind it doesn't make the problem go away. For that you need a tool like EFT.

Since its beginnings, EFT has improved the golf swings, tennis backhands, springboard dives, batting averages, bowling scores, and gymnastic moves of men, women, and children around the globe. Now EFT has begun moving from the realm of anecdotal reports into the world of scientific investigation.

In May 2008, Dawson Church, Ph.D., presented a paper at the tenth annual conference of the Association for Comprehensive Energy Psychology, or ACEP, titled "The Effect of Energy Psychology on Athletic Performance: A Randomized Controlled Blind Trial." He reported on the first-ever study of athletic performance and EFT. The study used a rigorous "randomized controlled" design, which is regarded as the Gold Standard of scientific proof. The study investigated whether EFT could affect athletic performance by evaluating whether a single brief EFT treatment for performance stress could produce an improvement in two skills for high-performance men's and women's college basketball teams at Oregon State University. The treatment group received a brief EFT session while the control group listened to basketball tips and techniques from an article written by former championship basketball coach Rick Pitino.

The performance of the players was measured on free throws and vertical jump height. Basketball players who received the EFT intervention scored an average of 21 percent better individually in free throws after treatment than the control group, while, at the end of a fatiguing two-hour basketball game, the control group scored an average that was 17 percent lower (p<0.028). The EFT group also jumped higher, though their improvement did not quite reach the threshold required for statistical significance, which is that there is one possibility in 20 that the results could be due to chance. These findings indicate that EFT performed as an intervention during the course of an athletic event may reduce performance stress and improve individual player function for free throws. The results of Church's ground-breaking experiment were published in *Open Sports Sciences*, a peer-reviewed psychology journal.

A later analysis of Church's Oregon State results by Harvey Baker, Ph.D. of Queens College in New York examined the results of the lowest-performing players who took part in the experiment. It excluded the highest-performing players because if a player entered the study already able to make 10 out of 10 baskets, no further improvement was possible. Baker found an even greater effect for EFT when the top performers were excluded. His analysis was published in the peer-reviewed journal *Energy Psychology: Theory, Research, & Treatment.*

In another Oregon State triumph for EFT, baseball coach Dan Spencer had therapist Greg Warburton, LPC, introduce EFT to Division 1 college baseball in the middle of the 2006 season. With key players using EFT, Oregon State went on to win the College Baseball World

Series in 2006 and then won an unprecedented second consecutive championship in 2007.

I look forward to seeing future studies published in peer-reviewed scientific and medical journals documenting the effectiveness of EFT not only for sports performance but for all of life's challenges.

Here, in the mean time, is your opportunity to learn a technique that is easy to understand, easy to use, and easy to share with others. EFT is fully portable—it's always with you and always available—and it can help improve almost any situation, no matter how challenging.

I would like to remind readers that EFT is a universal healing aid. That is, the same basic formula works for just about any condition. You will use the same procedure to get rid of a headache, improve a relationship, increase your income, overcome an illness, break an old habit, or improve your coordination. If you're a golfer, you may be tempted to read only golf-related reports in the examples that follow, but I hope you'll read everything. It may be that your sports performance problem has more in common with one of our EFT bowling stories than it does with the golf reports, or vice versa. The same is true for players of all the games mentioned here. In EFT workshops and seminars, people routinely tap for problems that seem to have nothing to do with them, yet they gain important insights and find their own situations improving dramatically.

This book is a general introduction to EFT for sports. I have also prepared an e-book supplement for golfers, titled *EFT for Golf.* I hope that in the future, other EFT coaches, practitioners, and players will describe EFT's applications to many different games and activities in books, e-books, workshops, and seminars. In the mean time, everything you need to start transforming your life and your game is here in these pages.

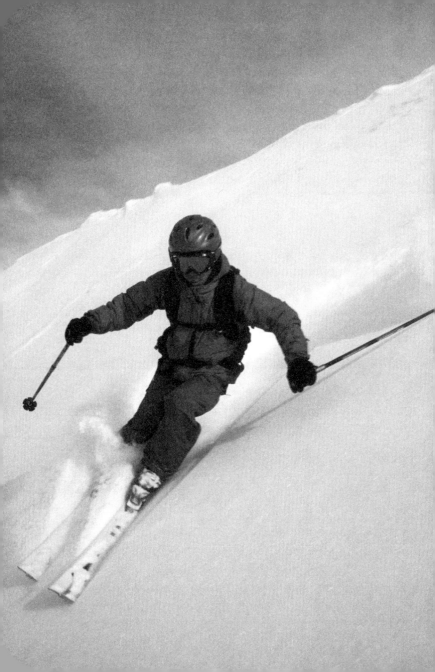

1

Getting Started

Welcome to EFT

The basic premise of the Emotional Freedom Techniques is that *the cause of all negative emotions is a disruption in the body's energy system.* I can't emphasize this concept enough. When our energy is flowing normally, without obstruction, we feel good in every way. When our energy becomes blocked or stagnant or is otherwise disrupted along one or more of the body's energy meridians, negative or damaging emotions can develop along with all types of physical symptoms. This idea has been the centerpiece of Eastern medicine for thousands of years.

EFT is often called *emotional acupuncture* because it combines gentle tapping on key acupuncture points while focusing your thoughts on pain, unhappy memories, uncomfortable emotions, food cravings, or any other problem. When properly done, the underlying emotional factors that contribute to the problem are typically released along with the energy blocks.

Consider that:

EFT often works when nothing else will.

- **Further, it can bring complete or partial relief in about 80 percent of the cases in which it's tried,** and in the hands of a skilled practitioner, its success rate can exceed 95 percent.

- **Sometimes the improvement is permanent,** while in other cases the process needs to be continued. But even if symptoms return, they can usually be reduced or eliminated quickly and effectively just by repeating the procedure.

- **People are often astonished at the results they experience** because their belief systems have not yet adapted to this common-sense process. The treatment of physical, emotional, and performance issues is supposed to be much more difficult than simply tapping with your fingertips on key acupuncture points.

- **The EFT basics are extremely easy to use.** Small children learn it quickly, and kids as young as eight or ten have no trouble teaching it to others. It's fully portable, requires no special equipment, and can be used at any time of the day or night and under any circumstances.

- **No drugs, surgeries, radiations, or other medical interventions** are involved in EFT. In fact, it's so different from conventional medicine that the medical profession often has difficulty explaining its results.

- **It doesn't seem to matter what the patient's blood tests or other diagnostic tests show.** Relief can occur with EFT no matter what your diagnosis. That's because we are addressing a different cause that tends to be outside the medical box.

- **This is not to say you should ignore your physician's advice.** On the contrary, I encourage you to consult with qualified health care providers. Quite a few EFT practitioners are physicians, nurses, dentists, acupuncturists, chiropractors, massage therapists, psychologists, counselors, and other health care professionals. As EFT becomes more widely known, it will become easier to find licensed health care providers who are knowledgeable about EFT.

- **Using a few minutes of EFT will often improve your physical health.** When it doesn't, there is likely to be some underlying emotional issue that is creating chemicals and/or tension in your body that interferes with your success.

- If that's the case, **EFT is ideal for collapsing and neutralizing emotional issues** and it often does the job in minutes. EFT was originally designed for reducing the psychotherapy process from months or years down to minutes or, in complicated cases, a few sessions.

No technique or procedure works for everyone but by all accounts the vast majority of those who try EFT for a specific problem experience significant improvement. That's a stunning result and one that compares favorably with prescription drugs, surgical procedures, and other medical treatments.

EFT is so new that it's still evolving. I encourage practitioners and newcomers alike to experiment—to try it on everything. It makes sense that if your energy is balanced, everything inside and around you benefits.

Whether you are new to EFT or already an experienced tapper, I am very pleased to share this information with you. I know without a doubt that EFT can help you take control of your health and happiness and that the instructions and recommendations given here can completely transform your life.

Defining the Problem

EFT sessions usually begin with a self-estimate of discomfort using a scale from zero to 10. We call this the 0-to-10 intensity meter or intensity scale. The discomfort being measured can be physical, such as headache pain or a craving, or it can be an emotion such as fear, anxiety, depression, or anger.

Intensity Meter

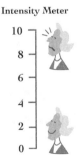

It's a good idea to rate every problem before and after you apply EFT so that you can determine how much progress you're making. It's also important to assess your intensity as it exists now rather than when the event or problem first occurred.

Don't worry if you find it difficult to select a specific number—sometimes newbies (my affectionate term for EFT newcomers) get distracted by this part of the procedure and worry unnecessarily about whether it's a 5 or a 6, or a 2 or a 3. Using the 10-point scale becomes easy with practice. Just give yourself a number to get started and it will soon be automatic. It helps to remind yourself that there are no wrong answers here and that if you have trouble coming up with a specific number, a guess will work fine. It is simply a benchmark for comparison before and after you perform EFT.

For reference, jot the number down and add a few notes. For example, if you're focusing on a pain, think about where the pain is located, how it interferes with your range of motion, and whether it hurts more when you move to the left or right, stand or sit, and so forth.

Another way to indicate the intensity of pain or discomfort that works well for children is by stretching one's arms wide apart for major pain and putting them close together for minor pain. Some children find it easier to express "big" and "small" with their hands than with a number scale.

The method you choose doesn't matter as long as it works for you. Keeping track of your pain's intensity before and after treatment is the easiest way to determine whether and how effectively the treatment is working.

The same scale works for feelings. First, focus on an event or memory or problem that has been bothering you. Now ask yourself how angry, anxious, depressed, or upset you are on a scale from zero to 10. If it doesn't bother you at all, you're at zero. If you're at 10, that's the most it has ever been. Get in the habit of starting each tapping session with an intensity measurement and make a note of it.

Now, borrowing some pages from *The EFT Manual*, I'd like to introduce you to the Basic Recipe, the formula that is the foundation of this technique.

The Basic Recipe

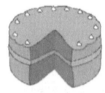

A recipe has certain ingredients that must be added in a certain order. If you are baking a cake, for example, you must use sugar instead of pepper and you must add the sugar *before* you put it in the oven. Otherwise… no cake.

Basic EFT is like a cake recipe. It has specific ingredients that go together in a specific way. Just as someone who is learning to cook will get best results from following tried and true instructions, someone who is new to EFT will do well to learn the Basic Recipe. An accomplished chef will take a different approach, and so can you once you master the fundamentals.

What I'm going to show you here is a shortcut method of using EFT. It does not include everything that

I teach in *The EFT Manual* or in the training materials at www.EFTUniverse.com. However, after developing EFT, I discovered that this shortcut method works very well almost all of the time, so this is the primary method I now use, and so do most EFT practitioners. I encourage everyone to learn or at least know about the original version so that if you don't get the results you want, you can try the complete Basic Recipe. It is easy to learn and adds less than a minute to the procedure. The complete Basic Recipe is explained in Appendix A of this book.

Focusing now on the shortcut method, here is what you need in order to start using EFT.

Ingredient #1: The Setup

Applying the Basic Recipe is something like going bowling. In bowling, there is a machine that sets up the pins by picking them up and arranging them in perfect order at the end of the alley. Once this "setup" is done, all you need to do is roll the ball down the alley to knock over the pins.

In a similar manner, the Basic Recipe has a beginning routine to "set up" your energy system as though it is a set of bowling pins. This routine (called the Setup) is vital to the whole process and prepares the energy system so that the rest of the Basic Recipe (the ball) can do its job.

Your energy system, of course, is not *really* a set of bowling pins. It is a set of subtle electric circuits. I present this bowling analogy only to give you a sense of the purpose of the Setup and the need to **make sure your**

energy system is properly oriented before attempting to remove its disruptions.

Your energy system is subject to a form of electrical interference which can block the balancing effect of these tapping procedures. When present, this interfering blockage must be removed or the Basic Recipe will not work. Removing it is the job of the Setup.

Technically speaking, this interfering blockage takes the form of a *polarity reversal* within your energy system. This is different from the *energy disruptions* that cause your negative emotions.

Another analogy may help us here. Consider a flashlight or any other device that runs on batteries. If the batteries aren't there, it won't work. Equally important, *the batteries must be installed properly.* You've noticed, I'm sure, that batteries have + and - marks on them. These marks indicate their *polarity.* If you line up the + and - marks according to the instructions, the electricity flows normally and your flashlight works fine.

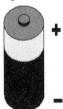

But what happens if you put the batteries in backwards? Try it sometime. The flashlight will not work. It acts as if the batteries have been removed. That's what happens when polarity reversal is present in your energy system. It's as though your batteries are in backwards.

I don't mean that you stop working altogether—like turn "toes up" and die—but your progress *does* become arrested in some areas.

Psychological Reversal

This polarity reversal has an official name. It is called Psychological Reversal and it represents a fascinating discovery with wide-ranging applications in **all areas of healing and personal performance.**

It is the reason why some diseases are chronic and respond very poorly to conventional treatments. It is the reason why some people have such a difficult time losing weight or giving up addictive substances. It is also the reason why talented athletes "freeze" or make game-losing mistakes or never achieve their full potential. It is, quite literally, the cause of self-sabotage.

Psychological Reversal is caused by self-defeating, negative thinking that often occurs subconsciously and thus outside of your awareness. On average, it will be present—and thus hinder EFT—about 40 percent of the time. Some people have very little of it (this is rare) while others are beset by it most of the time (this also is rare). Most people fall somewhere in between these two extremes. Psychological reversal doesn't create any feelings within you so you won't know if it is present or not. Even the most positive people are subject to it...including yours truly.

When psychological reversal is present, it will stop any attempt at healing, including EFT, dead in its tracks.

Therefore **it <u>must</u> be corrected if the rest of the Basic Recipe is going to work.**

We correct for Psychological Reversal *even though it might not be present.* It only takes 8 or 10 seconds to do and, if it isn't present, no harm is done. If it *is* present, however, a major impediment to your success will be out of the way.

The Setup consists of two parts, which are:

1) saying an affirmation three times and

2) simultaneously correcting for Psychological Reversal.

The Affirmation

Since the cause of Psychological Reversal involves negative thinking, it should come as no surprise that the correction for it includes a neutralizing affirmation. Such is the case with EFT, and here it is.

Even though I have this _____, I deeply and completely accept myself.

Fill in the blank with a brief description of the problem you want to address. Here are some examples.

Even though I have this <u>pain in my lower back</u>, I deeply and completely accept myself.

Even though I have this <u>fear of public speaking</u>, I deeply and completely accept myself.

Even though I have this <u>headache</u>, I deeply and completely accept myself.

Even though I have this <u>anger towards my father</u>, I deeply and completely accept myself.

Even though I have this <u>war memory</u>, I deeply and completely accept myself.

Even though I have this <u>stiffness in my neck</u>, I deeply and completely accept myself.

Even though I have these <u>nightmares</u>, I deeply and completely accept myself.

Even though I have this <u>craving for chocolate</u>, I deeply and completely accept myself.

Even though I have this <u>fear of snakes</u>, I deeply and completely accept myself.

This is only a partial list, of course, because the possible issues that are addressable by EFT are endless. You can also vary the acceptance phrase by saying:

"I accept myself even though I have this _____."

"Even though I have this _____, I deeply and profoundly accept myself."

"Even though _____, I love and forgive myself."

"I love and accept myself even though I have this _____."

And there are more variations. Instead of saying, "I deeply and completely accept myself," you can simply say:

I'm OK.	*I'll be OK.*
I'll feel better soon.	*Everything's improving.*

Or something similar. This, by the way, is how we use EFT with children. The phrase "I deeply and completely accept myself" makes little sense to kids. Instead, a child who's upset can say something like the following:

Even though I flunked the math test, I'm a cool kid, I'm OK.

Even though I lost my backpack and I'm mad at myself, I'm still an awesome kid.

All of these affirmations are correct because they follow the same general format. That is, they acknowledge the problem and create self-acceptance despite the existence of the problem.

That's what is necessary for the affirmation to be effective. You can use any version, but I suggest you start with the recommended one because it is easy to memorize and has a good track record of getting the job done.

Now here are some interesting points about the affirmation:

- It doesn't matter whether you believe the affirmation or not. Just say it.

- It is better to say it with feeling and emphasis, but saying it routinely will usually do the job.

- It is best to say it out loud, but if you are in a social situation where you prefer to mutter it under your breath or do it silently, then go ahead. It will probably be effective.

Correcting for Psychological Reversal

To add to the effectiveness of the affirmation, the Setup includes a simple method for clearing Psychological

Reversal. You do this by tapping the Karate Chop point, which is explained next, while reciting the affirmation.

The Karate Chop Point

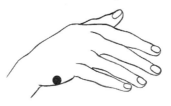

The Karate Chop (KC) Point

The Karate Chop point (abbreviated **KC**) is located at the center of the fleshy part of the outside of your hand (either hand) between the top of the wrist and the base of the baby finger—or, stated differently, the part of your hand you would use to deliver a karate chop.

Solidly tap the Karate Chop point with the tips of the index finger and middle finger—or all four fingers—of the opposite hand. While you *could* use the Karate Chop point of either hand, it is usually most convenient to tap the Karate Chop point of the non-dominant hand with the fingertips of the dominant hand. If you are right-handed, tap the Karate Chop point on your left hand with the fingertips of your right hand. If you are left-handed, tap the Karate Chop point on your right hand with the fingertips of your left hand.

Now that you understand the parts of the Setup, performing it is easy. You create a word or short phrase to fill in the blank in the affirmation and then **simply repeat the**

affirmation, with emphasis, three times while continuously tapping the Karate Chop point.

That's it. After a few practice rounds, you should be able to perform the Setup in eight to ten seconds or so. Now, with the Setup properly performed, you are ready for the next ingredient in the Basic Recipe—the Sequence.

Ingredient #2: The Sequence

The Sequence is very simple in concept. It involves tapping at or near the end points of the body's major energy flows, which are called *meridians* in Oriental medicine, and it is the method by which the disruption in the energy system is corrected or balanced out. Before locating these points, however, you need a few tips on how to carry out the tapping process.

Tapping tips: You can tap with either hand or both hands but it is usually more convenient to do so with your dominant hand (your right hand if you are right-handed or your left hand if you are left-handed).

Tap with the fingertips of your index finger and middle finger. This covers a little larger area than just tapping with one fingertip and allows you to cover the tapping points more easily.

Tap solidly but never so hard as to hurt or bruise yourself.

Tap about seven times on each of the tapping points. I say about seven times because you will be repeating a "Reminder Phrase" (explained later) while tapping and it will be difficult to count at the same time. If you are a little over or a little under seven (five to nine, for example) that will be sufficient.

Most of the tapping points exist on either side of the body. It doesn't matter which side you use nor does it matter if you switch sides during the Sequence. For example, you can tap under your right eye and, later in the Sequence, tap under your left arm.

The points: Each energy meridian has two end points. For the purposes of the Basic Recipe, you need only tap on one end point to balance out any disruptions that may exist in the meridian. These end points are near the surface of the body and are thus more readily accessed than other points along the meridians that may be more deeply buried. What follows are instructions on how to locate the end points of those meridians that are important to the Basic Recipe. Taken together and done in the order presented, they form the Sequence.

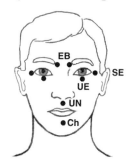

EB, SE, UE, UN and Ch Points

Eyebrow: At the beginning of the eyebrow, just above and to one side of the nose. This point is abbreviated **EB** for beginning of the **E**ye**B**row.

Side of Eye: On the bone bordering the outside corner of the eye. This point is abbreviated **SE** for **S**ide of the **E**ye.

Under Eye: On the bone under an eye about 1 inch below the pupil. This point is abbreviated **UE** for **U**nder the **E**ye.

Under Nose: On the small area between the bottom of the nose and the top of the upper lip. This point is abbreviated **UN** for **U**nder the **N**ose.

Chin: Midway between the point of your chin and the bottom of your lower lip. Although it is not directly on the point of the chin, we call it the Chin Point because it is descriptive enough for people to understand easily. This point is abbreviated **Ch** for **Ch**in.

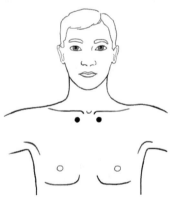

The Collarbone (CB) Points

Collarbone: The junction where the sternum (breastbone), collarbone, and first rib meet. Place your forefinger on the U-shaped notch at the top of the breastbone (where a man would knot his tie). Move down toward the navel 1 inch and then go to the left (or right) 1 to 2 inches. This point is abbreviated **CB** for **C**ollar**B**one *even though it is not on the collarbone (or clavicle) per se.* It is at the *beginning* of the collarbone.

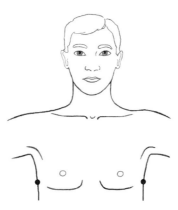

The Underarm (UA) Points

Underarm: On the side of the body, at a point even with the nipple (for men) or in the middle of the bra strap (for women). It is about 4 inches below the armpit. This point is abbreviated **UA** for **U**nder the **A**rm.

The abbreviations for these points are summarized in the same order as given above.

EB = Beginning of the **E**ye**B**row

SE = **S**ide of the **E**ye

UE = **U**nder the **E**ye

UN = **U**nder the **N**ose

Ch = **Ch**in

CB = Beginning of the **CollarBone**

UA = Under the **Arm**

Please notice that these tapping points proceed *down the body.* That is, each tapping point is *below* the one before it. That should make it a snap to memorize. A few trips through it and it should be yours forever.

The Reminder Phrase

Once memorized, the Basic Recipe becomes a lifetime friend. It can be applied to an almost endless list of emotional and physical problems, and it provides relief from most of them. However, there's one more concept we need to develop before we can apply the Basic Recipe to a given problem. It's called the Reminder Phrase.

When a football quarterback throws a pass, he aims it at a particular receiver. He doesn't just throw the ball in the air and hope someone will catch it. Likewise, the Basic Recipe needs to be aimed at a specific problem. Otherwise, it will bounce around aimlessly with little or no effect.

You "aim" the Basic Recipe by applying it while "tuned in" to the problem from which you want relief. This tells your system which problem needs to be the receiver.

Remember the EFT discovery statement, which says: *The cause of all negative emotions is a disruption in the body's energy system.*

Negative emotions come about because you are tuned into certain thoughts or circumstances that, in turn, disrupt your energy system. Otherwise, you function nor-mally. One's fear of heights is not present, for example, while one is reading the comic section of the Sunday newspaper and therefore not tuned in to the problem.

Tuning in to a problem can be done by simply think-ing about it. In fact, tuning in *means* thinking about it. Thinking about the problem will bring about the energy disruptions involved, which then and only then, can be balanced by applying the Basic Recipe. Without tuning in to the problem—thereby creating those energy disrup-tions—the Basic Recipe does nothing.

Tuning in is seemingly a very simple process. You merely think about the problem while applying the Basic Recipe. That's it, at least in theory.

However, you may find it a bit difficult to consciously think about the problem while you are tapping. That's why I'm introducing a Reminder Phrase that you can repeat continually while performing the Basic Recipe.

The Reminder Phrase is simply a word or short phrase that describes the problem and that you repeat out loud each time you tap one of the points in the Sequence. In this way you continually "remind" your system about the problem you are working on.

The best Reminder Phrase to use is usually identical to what you choose for the affirmation part of the Setup. For example, if you are working on a fear of public speak-ing, the Setup affirmation would go like this:

Even though I have this <u>fear of public speaking</u>, I deeply and completely accept myself.

Within this affirmation, the underlined words, *fear of public speaking,* are ideal for use as the Reminder Phrase.

I sometimes use a shorter version of this Reminder Phrase when in seminars. I might, for example, use "public speaking fear" or just "public speaking" instead of the somewhat longer version shown above. That's just one of the shortcuts we have grown accustomed to after years of experience with these techniques. For your purposes, however, you can simply use identical words for both the Setup's affirmation and the Reminder Phrase. That way you will minimize any possibility for error.

Now here's an interesting point. *I don't always have people repeat a Reminder Phrase.* That's because I have discovered over time that simply stating the affirmation during the Setup is usually sufficient to "tune in" to the problem at hand. The subconscious mind usually locks on to the problem throughout the Basic Recipe even though tapping might seem distracting.

But this is not always true and, with extensive training and experience, one can recognize whether or not using the Reminder Phrase is necessary. As stated, it is not usually necessary, but *when it is necessary it is really necessary and must be used.*

What's beautiful about EFT is that you don't need to have my experience in this regard. You don't have to be able to figure out whether or not the Reminder Phrase is necessary. You can just *assume* it is always necessary and thereby assure yourself of always being tuned in to the problem by simply repeating the Reminder Phrase as instructed. It does no harm to repeat the Reminder

Phrase when it is not necessary, and it will serve as an invaluable tool when it is. We do many things in each round of the Basic Recipe that may not be necessary for a given problem. But when a particular part of the Basic Recipe is necessary, *it is absolutely critical.*

It does no harm to include everything, even what may not be needed, and *it only takes one minute per round.* This includes *always* repeating the Reminder Phrase each time you tap a point during the Sequence. It costs nothing to include it, not even time, because it can be repeated within the same time it takes to tap each energy point seven times.

This concept about the Reminder Phrase is an easy one. But just to be complete, I am including a few samples:

headache	*nightmares*
anger towards my father	*craving for chocolate*
war memory	*fear of snakes*
stiffness in my neck	

Test Your Results

At the end of one or two rounds of tapping all of the points in the Sequence, take another look at the problem you're working on. Measure it on the 0-to-10 intensity scale. Where is it now? You'll be able to test some problems or conditions right away, in the comfort of your living room. Others you'll want to test in the actual settings where they occur.

If the problem doesn't bother you at all any more and is at zero, congratulations. You're done. No further tapping is required.

If you feel better but the problem is still there, make a note of your new level of discomfort on the 0-to-10 intensity scale. For example, your headache pain may have gone from a 9 to a 4, or your anger toward your father might have moved from an 8 to a 5. Keeping track of the numbers helps you keep track of your progress.

If you are a practitioner, write down the problem your client is working on, the beginning intensity level, and the level after treatment. This helps both of you appreciate whatever improvement is being made, and it simplifies follow-up sessions.

If you're working on your own, write down every problem or issue you tap for along with your results. Review your notes after a few weeks of practice and you will be amazed at the number of issues you have cleared away, many of which you will have forgotten about by then.

Here's what to do if you or your client still have some discomfort after an initial round of tapping.

Subsequent-round Adjustments

When EFT tapping produces only partial relief, you will need to do one or more additional rounds.

Those subsequent rounds have to be adjusted slightly for best results. Here's why. The first round doesn't always completely eliminate a problem because of the re-emergence of Psychological Reversal, that interfering blockage that the Setup is designed to correct.

This time, Psychological Reversal shows up in a somewhat different form. Instead of blocking your progress altogether, it now blocks any *remaining* progress. You make some headway but become stopped on the way to complete relief because Psychological Reversal enters in a manner that keeps you from *getting any better still.*

Since the subconscious mind tends to be very literal, subsequent rounds of the Basic Recipe need to address the fact that you are working on the *remaining problem.* Accordingly, the affirmation contained within the Setup has to be adjusted, as does the Reminder Phrase.

> *Even though I **still** have **some of** this* _____, *I deeply and completely accept myself.*

Please note the emphasized words (***still*** and ***some of***) and how they change the thrust of the affirmation toward the *remainder* of the problem. It should be easy to make this adjustment and, after a little experience, you will fall into it quite naturally.

Study the affirmations below. They reflect adjustments to the affirmations shown earlier in this section.

> *Even though I **still** have **some of** this <u>headache</u>, I deeply and completely accept myself.*

> *Even though I **still** have **some of** this <u>anger towards my father</u>, I deeply and completely accept myself.*

> *Even though I **still** have **some of** this <u>war memory</u>, I deeply and completely accept myself.*

*Even though I **still** have **some of** this <u>stiffness in my neck</u>, I deeply and completely accept myself.*

The Reminder Phrase is also easily adjusted. Just put the word *"remaining"* before the previously used phrase. Here, as examples, are the previous Reminder Phrases:

remaining *headache*

remaining *anger towards my father*

remaining *war memory*

remaining *stiffness in my neck*

If your symptom or condition disappears but then returns, simply repeat EFT's Basic Recipe and the "remaining" Reminder Phrase described above.

Tapping with and for Others

I should add that EFT can be done by you on yourself, by another person on you, and by you on another person. All of these approaches to EFT tapping work equally well. If you watch my EFT sessions on my DVDs, you will see that in seminars and workshops, I routinely tap on the EFT points of the people I work with onstage.

The technique of tapping on another person makes it easy for parents to apply EFT to their infants and small children and for anyone to apply EFT to those who for various reasons are not able to tap on or for themselves.

Introducing Aspects

Aspects are the various pieces of an emotional issue that may show up during an EFT session. Fortunately, they can be handled easily.

For example, let's say you have a fear of spiders that you would like to put behind you. If there is no spider present to cause you any emotional intensity, then close your eyes and imagine seeing a spider, or imagine a past time when a spider scared you. Assess your intensity on a scale of 0 to 10 *as it exists NOW while you think about it.* If you estimate it at a 7, for example, then you have a benchmark against which to measure your progress.

Now do one round of the Basic Recipe and imagine the spider again. If you can find no trace whatsoever of your previous emotional intensity, then you are done. If, on the other hand, you go to, let's say, a 4, then you need to perform subsequent rounds until your intensity falls to zero.

You might wonder at this point whether getting to zero while just *thinking* about a spider will hold up when you actually confront a real spider. The answer is usually *yes!* In most cases, the energy disruptions that occur while *thinking* about the spider are the same as those that occur when you are in the presence of a real spider. That's why the original energy balancing tends to hold in real circumstances.

The exception to this is when some new aspect of the problem comes up in the real situation that wasn't there when you were just thinking about it. For example, you may have been *thinking* about a stationary spider that didn't move. If movement is an important aspect of your fear and if it was absent from your thinking when the original EFT rounds were done, then that part of the fear will arise when you see a moving spider.

This is a reasonably common occurrence and *it doesn't mean that EFT didn't work.* It simply means there is more to do. Just apply the Basic Recipe to the new aspect (moving spider) until your emotional response falls to zero. Once all aspects have been eliminated, your phobic response to spiders should be history and you can be perfectly calm around them.

Someone who's haunted by a traffic accident might be affected by memories of oncoming headlights, anger toward the other driver, the sound of screeching brakes, or the sight of window glass shattering. A war trauma can have aspects such as the sight of blood, the look in a comrade's eyes before he dies, the sound of a hand grenade, or the memory of an explosion or gunfire. A rape experience can have aspects such as the smell of the assailant's breath, the sound of his voice, the impact of a fist, the penetration, etc. A fear of public speaking can have aspects such as the sight of a microphone, the on-looking eyes of the audience, or a memory of being ridiculed as a child.

Another thing to recognize is that an aspect can also be an emotion. Some clients report that the anger they had regarding a given event has shifted to sadness. Pick up on these clues. These different emotional aspects are taking you deeper into the problem. They are opportunities for greater healing and present you with great possibilities for mastering your craft.

The notion of aspects is an important one in EFT. As in the examples above, some problems have many pieces or aspects to them and the problem will not be completely relieved until all of them are addressed. Actually, each of these aspects qualifies as a separate problem even though they seem to be all lumped together. The fear of a stationary spider and the fear of a moving spider, for example, would seem to be lumped together. In fact, they are separate problems that need to be addressed separately with EFT.

Different aspects are possible with just about any problem you want to address with EFT. Each aspect may be a separate problem that needs to be addressed individually before complete relief is obtained.

Please understand that where several aspects of an *emotional* problem are present, you may not notice any relief until all aspects are reduced to zero by the Basic Recipe. This becomes very clear when you consider different aspects of *physical* healing. If, for example, you have a simultaneous headache, toothache, and stomach ache, you will not feel healthy until all three are gone. The pain may seem to shift but it is, nonetheless, still pain. So it is with *emotional* issues that contain different aspects. Even if you have taken care of one or more aspects, you may not experience relief until all of the problem's aspects have been dealt with.

Experienced EFT'ers often compare this procedure to peeling an onion. You get rid of one layer only to discover another. When a problem has many layers or aspects, neutralizing them with EFT can seem like a daunting project. But considering how quickly those layers can be dealt with and how beneficial the results are, the project is more exciting than intimidating. And the rewards are priceless.

Core Issues

By far the fastest way to resolve a complex issue or clear up symptoms that resist treatment is to discover the problem's core issue. Core issues are fundamental emotional disruptions that can be formed in childhood or in response to a difficult or traumatic event.

In some cases they are obvious. When asked about when a problem started or what might be contributing to it, the reply is immediate. "I'll bet it has something to do with my husband's heart attack last fall." "I turn to food whenever I think about my wife's affair, and my overeating is out of control." "Ever since my business failed, my back has been killing me."

But many times, core issues are hidden from view. This is because the subconscious mind is a clever protector of secrets, especially those that we hide from ourselves.

In some cases, our subconscious minds hide secrets that are truly awful. But most self-sabotaging secrets, when looked at objectively, don't amount to much.

The reason Tom can't give a presentation at work is because in fourth grade, his teacher embarrassed him in front of the class. The reason Ann can't lose weight is because, when she was eight years old, her mother told her she would always be too fat to wear a swim suit. The reason John can't propose to Marie is because his older sister always told him that he was such a loser, no one would ever marry him. The reason Susan can't take an elevator is because when she was trapped in one for five minutes several years ago, the friend who was with her started screaming.

As long as they hold an emotional charge, these secrets are powerful enough to shape a person's life—but as soon as they are uncovered and neutralized with EFT, core issues like these lose their power and become insignificant old memories.

This feature of EFT never ceases to amaze me. Again and again I've worked with people while they dealt with incredibly painful memories, memories that controlled their lives and dictated where they would live, what career they would follow, what friends they would have, and everything else. Suddenly, after a few rounds of EFT tapping, they are completely transformed and no longer frightened, anxious, or afraid of old events. Instead, they're able to describe past traumas as easily as if they are talking about the weather. As soon as old events and old memories lose their emotional charge, they lose their place of power in the subconscious mind.

Be Specific

If you want fast, impressive results with EFT, be specific. Vague statements generate vague outcomes. The biggest mistake made by newcomers is using EFT on issues that are too global. Global problems are broad, vague, or hazy. They aren't well defined. Even with persistence, which can almost always make a difference, global statements are less likely to produce results than specific statements about specific events.

I have been beating the drum for many years about being specific with EFT, urging EFT'ers to break emotional issues into the events that underlie them. When we do this, we address true causes and not just symptoms. While there is a skill to doing this, those who take this approach have watched their success rates climb impressively. They are also doing deeper, more meaningful work.

Many newcomers to EFT present their emotional issues in very global terms. They say things like:

I feel abandoned. I'm always anxious.

I was an abused child. I hate my father.

I have low self-esteem. I can't do anything right.

I'm depressed. I feel overwhelmed.

To them, *that* is the problem and *that* is what they want EFT to fix.

But, despite the person's perception, that is not the problem at all. Those feelings are merely symptoms of the problem. The real problem is the unresolved specific events, memories, and emotions that cause the larger issue. How can one feel abandoned or abused, for example, unless specific events occurred in one's life to cause those feelings? The feelings didn't just appear out of the blue. They must have had a cause.

If we consider the larger issue (such as abandonment) to be a table top, then the table's legs represent specific events that support the table (my mother died when I was seven; my father walked out on us when I was eleven; I got lost on a hiking trip in the Sierra Mountains; etc.). Obviously, if we reduce an issue to the specific events supporting it and then collapse its table legs, the table top will fall for lack of support. In this way we address the true causes (specific events and emotions linked to them) rather than just symptoms.

Unfortunately, many EFT practitioners still apply EFT to the table top and not the supporting table legs. Thus they might start with…

Even though I have this feeling of abandonment…

Being too global like this is the number-one error made by new EFT'ers and some seasoned ones, too. Interestingly, this approach will sometimes get results but it is not nearly as thorough or precise as going for the supporting table legs first.

Also, because this global approach lacks precision, those using it are more likely to report that their issues "come back." What "come back," of course, are unresolved events (table legs) that were not previously addressed.

In addition, approaching an issue in a vague or global manner creates an environment in which the person's attention shifts from event to event. You can be much more accurate and achieve greater success if you reduce those global issues (table tops) to the specific events (table legs) that cause them. Examples for the global issue of "I feel abandoned" could include:

The time my mother left me in the shopping mall when I was in second grade.

The time my father told me to leave home when I was twelve.

The time my third-grade teacher gave me that "I don't care about you" look.

These specific events are much easier to deal with than the global issues they created. If you deal with them one at a time without letting your attention shift, it will be easy to clear them—and by clearing the emotions stored in these small specific events, you can automatically repair the larger global issue.

To this point, I have provided more general examples like "fear of public speaking," "these nightmares," or "this anxiety." As a beginner, you can learn the process using general phrases like this, and your system will address the specifics behind the scenes. However, to be more direct and get more powerful results, it's better to break those general issues into the specific events that are contributing to them.

For "these nightmares," simply take one nightmare at a time, or identify a difficult event that occurred around the time the nightmares began. For "fear of public speaking," make a list of all the events in which public speaking was uncomfortable for you and tap them away one by one. For issues like anxiety, stress, or depression, you are usually dealing with a combination of emotions so it may take a little longer to see significant results, but you can start by finding the past events that have upset you the most and address them with EFT.

For additional help in finding specific events to tap on, ask yourself questions like:

When did this problem start? What was I doing at the time? What was going on in my life?

What does this issue remind me of?

The Generalization Effect

That being said, I want to acquaint you now with a fascinating feature of EFT. I call it the Generalization Effect because, after you address a few related problems with EFT, the process starts to *generalize* over all those problems. For example, someone who has 100 traumatic memories of being abused usually finds that **after using EFT and neutralizing only five or ten of them, they *all* vanish.**

This is startling to some people because they have so many traumas in their life, they think they are in for unending sessions with these techniques. Not so — at least not usually. EFT often clears out a whole forest after cutting down just a few trees. You'll see an excellent example of this Generalization Effect in my session with Rich, the first veteran on the "Six Days at the VA" video at www. EFTUniverse.com.

The Movie Technique and Story Technique

When addressing specific events with EFT, we often use the Movie Technique or the Tell the Story Technique. In both methods, you review a past event while tapping to reduce its emotional charge. The difference between the two is that in the Movie Technique, you watch events unfold in your mind, as though you're watching a movie, while in the Tell the Story Technique, you describe the events aloud.

The "plot" of the movie or story is usually very short. If not, reduce the length down to one or two emotional crescendos because that sets up the target for EFT's aim. However, if jumping straight to the key event is too painful, the movie or story can begin a few minutes before the first emotional crescendo. The event may have hurt, but its retelling doesn't have to.

Unlike psychotherapy techniques that require clients to relive unpleasant past events in excruciating detail, EFT's approach is gentle and flexible. You watch the movie or tell the story until you reach a point that feels uncomfortable. Instead of forcing yourself to push on, just tap until the emotional intensity of that segment fades. When you feel comfortable again, resume the movie or story. When feelings rise up again, tap until they subside. Eventually you will be able to narrate the whole story without any emotional intensity and regain your freedom with respect to that memory.

Our bodies store traumas, and our mental movies are keys that unlock emotions that are stored with those traumas. Because EFT tapping reduces the emotional charge attached to past events, it transforms the traumas, memories, energy blocks, targeted body parts, and emotions that were previously locked together. With the emotional charge gone, the traumas become normal memories, the connections disappear, and the pain once associated with them vanishes as well.

EFT's Constricted Breathing Technique

The Constricted Breathing Technique is a breathing exercise enhanced by tapping which, despite its simplicity, offers numerous benefits. It is a popular demonstration in workshops and client sessions because most people have constricted breathing and it is eye-opening to experience the improvements that EFT generates in a minute or two. Increased oxygen levels are so important to health that practically everyone who tries this procedure feels better as a result. Daily use can help improve physical fitness, and because it's relaxing, the technique is an attitude-adjustment tool that can help you move from stressed or anxious to calm and serene in record time. This makes it an effective aid to performance improvement as well as setting and reaching any new goal.

To use the technique, take two or three deep breaths. Take your time and don't hyperventilate. This step will stretch your lungs so that any EFT improvement in your breathing will not result from a normal "stretching effect."

Once you have stretched your lungs as far as they will go, take another deep breath. This time assess the deepness of your breath on a 0-to-10 scale, where 10 is your estimate of your maximum capacity. Most people start with numbers from 3 to 9. Those who rate their breath at a 10 (they are usually wrong) may find that after EFT they will go to a 12 or 15.

Now do several rounds of EFT with Setup Phrases such as:

> *Even though my breathing is constricted, I deeply and completely accept myself.*
>
> *Even though I can only fill my lungs to an 8...*
>
> *Even though I'm not used to breathing deeply...*

and so on. Be sure to include any physical or medical condition that could interfere, such as:

> *Even though I'm coming down with a cold [or have allergies or emphysema or a bruised rib] and it's hard to breathe, I deeply and completely accept myself.*

After each round, take another deep breath and assess your 0-to-10 lung capacity. In the vast majority of cases it will keep expanding and improving.

To clear any emotional cause of constricted or shallow breathing, ask yourself:

> *What does this constricted breath remind me of?*
>
> *When have I felt constricted or smothered?*
>
> *If there was an emotional reason for my constricted breath, what might it be?*

Often, these questions give big clues to important emotional issues. With the help of the Constricted Breathing Technique, whatever you feel upset, distressed, angry, disappointed, frustrated, guilty, irritated, sad, uncomfortable, or unhappy about can be more easily identified, incorporated into an EFT Setup Phrase, and tapped for.

Secondary Gain

Secondary gain is a psychiatric term meaning that the person has a reason for holding onto an undesirable condition, even though he or she may not recognize it.

The term applies to a wide variety of issues. An example would be chronic pain cases in which the patient will lose certain benefits by getting well, such as attention from others, monetary compensation for disability, or the ability to keep denying the original cause of the pain.

In metaphysics, the term "secondary gain" helps explain why we seem to run into barriers when it comes to manifesting our good. This occurs when we put a great deal of energy into visualizing, affirming, and treating for a new level of good and it either doesn't happen or the situation actually gets worse. The subconscious mind feels more secure in the disadvantaged state than in going for improvement. So while your conscious mind might be saying, *"I sincerely want to get over this problem,"* your subconscious screams, *"No, I don't!"*

If you suspect secondary gain, consider the following:

> *What benefits do you receive from your problem?*
> *Does keeping the problem feel safe?*
> *Does releasing it feel dangerous?*

Does keeping the problem generate sympathy from others that you won't receive if you release the problem?

Does keeping the problem allow you to avoid unpleasant situations?

Does keeping the problem give you financial rewards that you won't receive without it?

Do you feel you don't deserve to get over the problem?

Do you fear that if you get better, something bad will happen?

Interestingly enough, secondary gain issues can be broken down into specific events, just like other issues. The process is more difficult because the problem is usually stated very globally or generally, but if you keep asking yourself *"Why?"* or *"What's behind that?"* you are likely to find some specific events to address.

The Personal Peace Procedure

In my online tutorial, I describe the *Personal Peace Procedure,* which is an easy exercise that can help you tap away your issues one event at a time. This is especially helpful if you are having trouble finding your core issues or if you just want something to tap on every day. Although you may not be targeting the core issue behind a specific problem every time, you will be able to clear a large volume of unresolved emotions in a relatively short period of time. This is a different approach from targeting only the issues that contribute to specific problems, but the end result is often more complete.

Try it now. The sooner you start, the sooner you'll experience true personal peace.

1. **Make a list.** On a blank sheet of paper or at your computer, make a list of every bothersome specific event you can remember. If you don't find at least 50, you are either going at this half-heartedly or you have been living on some other planet. Many people find hundreds.

2. **List everything.** While making your list you may find that some events don't seem to cause you any current discomfort. That's OK. List them anyway. The mere fact that you remember them suggests a need for resolution.

3. **Give each event a title** as though it is a mini-movie. Examples:

   Dad hit me in the kitchen.

   I stole Suzie's sandwich.

   I almost slipped and fell into the Grand Canyon.

   My third grade class ridiculed me when I gave that speech.

   Mom locked me in a closet for hours.

   Mrs. Adams told me I was stupid.

4. **Tap for the big ones.** When the list is complete, pick out the biggest redwoods in your negative forest (the ones closest to 10 on the 0-to-10 scale) and apply EFT to each one of them until you either laugh about it or just can't think about it any more. Be sure to

notice any aspects that may come up and consider them separate trees in your negative forest. Apply EFT to them accordingly. Be sure to keep after each event until it is resolved down to zero. After the biggest redwoods are removed, look for the next-biggest, etc.

5. **Work on at least one movie per day**—preferably three—for three months. It takes only minutes per day. At this rate you will resolve 90 to 270 specific events in three months. Then notice how your body feels better. Note, too, how your threshold for getting upset is much lower. Note how your relationships are better and how many of your therapy-type issues just don't seem to be there any more. Revisit some specific events and notice how those previously intense incidents have faded into nothingness. Note any improvements in your life.

I ask you to consciously notice these things because, unless you do, the quality healing you will have undergone may be so subtle that you don't notice it. You may even dismiss it by saying, "Oh well, it was never much of a problem anyway." This happens repeatedly with EFT and thus I bring it to your awareness.

6. **If necessary, see your physician.** If you are taking prescription medications, you may feel the need to discontinue them. Please do so only under the supervision of a qualified health care practitioner.

It is my hope that the Personal Peace Procedure will become a worldwide routine. A few minutes per day will make a monumental difference in school performance, the workplace, relationships, health, and our quality of life. But these are meaningless words unless you put the idea into practice. As my good friend Howard Wight says, "If you are ultimately going to do something important that will make a real difference…do it now."

Is EFT Working Yet?

Whenever EFT produces dramatic results, the changes are obvious. You start out afraid of heights and now you're comfortable leaning over a fire escape or climbing a ladder. You had a migraine headache and now you feel terrific. You were mad at your boss and now you're laughing.

But not every improvement occurs right away. Sometimes nothing seems to happen during your tapping session and you give up in disappointment—but then a few hours later or the following day, you notice that the problem has completely disappeared. EFT can have a delayed effect.

And not all improvements are obvious. Some occur so subtly that they are barely noticed or not noticed at all. Paying attention to all aspects of your life, not just the symptoms you are treating with EFT, will help you appreciate these subtle results.

In a case reported by EFT practitioner Chrissie Hardisty, a 21-year-old client dropped out of college because of severe depression that did not respond to prescription anti-depressants. Fortunately, it did respond to tapping, and as the client later reported, his lifelong spider phobia disappeared as well. Spiders didn't enter his mind during his tapping session, and he only noticed this profound change of attitude when his father called it to his attention. Instead of having a panic attack at the sight of a spider, he remained calm and relaxed.

June Campbell used EFT to help her friend Betty overcome her fear of flying. As a bonus, Betty's severe dental pain, which had not responded to pain killers, disappeared during the session. "Betty hadn't mentioned the pain so I hadn't addressed it during tapping," she says. "The stubborn dental pain was gone as if by magic. That was two days ago. The pain has not returned. Betty is not at all anxious about her upcoming flight, and she reports having a better night's sleep than she's had in quite some time."

EFT practitioner Margo Arrowsmith worked with a man who was afraid of banks. After tapping away this fear with EFT, he was not only able to go into and out of banks with ease, but his sinus congestion—which he hadn't mentioned or addressed—disappeared for the first time in years. She says, "I have worked with people for their feelings of guilt about some minor childhood incident, and their headaches disappeared. Talk to any EFT practitioners and they will tell you lots of stories of unexpected and delightful side effects."

How might EFT tapping affect you? Individual results vary, but we have seen many situations in which EFT corrects problems that were not addressed or even thought of during the tapping. These results include:

relief from insomnia	*lower stress levels*
improved digestion	*increasing patience*
fewer headaches	*a more relaxed attitude*
better overall health	*more energy*
improved range of motion	*better relationships*
higher confidence levels	*increased efficiency*
improved memory	*growing optimism*
a reduction of fears and phobias	*relief from worry*
faster healing from illness or injury	*and more!*

Many of these changes could be overlooked if you aren't watching for them. Although there are many ways to keep track of the improvements EFT produces, one of the simplest is to make a list of your life's situations, your physical symptoms, and your feelings. Spend a few minutes each day or each week reviewing that list. Keeping a journal, diary, or notebook will help you remember details that might otherwise go unnoticed. Pay attention to the observations of others, too. They are evidence of transformations taking place within you.

This inventory is especially important if it seems as though EFT is not working. If you can't seem to release your emotional intensity, you still have an out-of-control craving, your elbow still hurts, you still feel depressed, or whatever you're addressing won't seem to budge, consider the possibility that other improvements are contributing to your success with the original problem.

In EFT, results can come quickly—or they can involve the repeated tapping sessions that we call "peeling the onion." You clear up one aspect of a problem only to have another appear, and it isn't until several of these layered aspects are dealt with that the problem completely goes away.

If it seems as though nothing is happening, don't give up. You might feel just as sad and discouraged as you did last week, but you may be sleeping better, or other drivers on the road don't annoy you the way they usually do. Your elbow may be as sore as it was yesterday, but you're criticizing your kids less and enjoying them more, or friends notice that you seem more relaxed. You're still helpless to resist chocolate ice cream, but you feel more energetic and complete a project at work ahead of schedule. Any of these or a thousand other small improvements suggest that your EFT tapping is producing deep-level changes.

Upcoming Examples

I have already described EFT as a flexible healing tool and, as you will see in this book, not all EFT sessions follow the basic instruction exactly.

This book includes an extensive collection of real stories about people who have used EFT for themselves or a friend, relative, client, or student for improved sports performance. These examples will help you understand how to use EFT in different situations, and how the basic principles you already know can be applied to an actual case—like yours.

I will provide plenty of narrative as we go so that you can see where the basic principles are being illustrated and where people have used their own variation to address a unique situation. Emotional issues are often complex, and there are many different ways to be specific or thorough with EFT. Accordingly, some people use fairly global or general approaches and others get all the way down to specific events, but they are all peeling away layers as they go.

One of the most obvious variations will be the extended Setup Phrases. With experience, you may find that using a longer description in the Setup to target your issue produces better results. By being more creative in the Setup you might trigger more memories than with the default or standard Setup, and that can help you get to deeper core issues.

One common misconception, however, is that the "right words" in the Setup are the magical key to results with EFT. This is not the case, although the examples you see in this book might leave you with that impression.

If you find that you "don't know what to say" in your Setup, you can always use the default or standard Setup Phrase, which is:

>   *Even though I have this _____, I deeply and completely accept myself.*

If you can't find a word for the _____, or if you aren't getting results, your Setup is probably too global, vague, or general, and you need to look deeper for a specific event related to the problem.

Once you find a specific event, use the Setup to describe it the same way you would tell it to a friend, and use the Tell the Story Technique to tap away the intensity one crescendo at a time. If addressing that event doesn't do the trick, then look for similar events, or try the Personal Peace Procedure.

Remember, getting results with EFT is more about *"What are you tapping for?"* than *"What words are you saying?"*

I encourage you to consider EFT a universal healing tool, something that can improve any and every part of your life. The more often you use it, the more likely you are to experience benefits in not just one or two areas but in all aspects of your being—and the more likely you are to completely resolve the original problem.

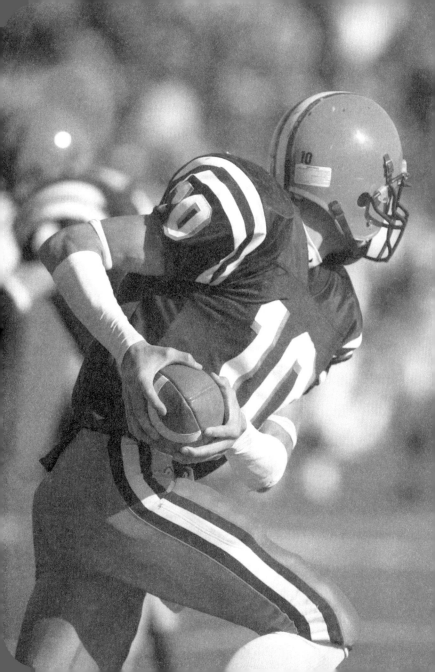

2

Better Sports
Performance

You don't have to be a sports psychologist to understand the adverse effects of stress, anxiety, and damaging self-talk in championship sports. Just watch a basketball playoff, a golf tournament, or the Olympics.

Now watch a growing number of professional and amateur athletes and coaches as they discover EFT and improve athletic accomplishments of every description. Tapping on key acupuncture points while focusing on the problem at hand balances the body's energy, eliminating fears and anxieties that interfere with performance.

Using EFT for performance issues is one of my favorite topics. Not only is it highly effective but it is also fun and rewarding. The results are often easy to recognize.

And for those with easily excited greed glands, there's a big financial potential when you apply EFT for business and sports performance. Businesses and professional sports teams pay big money for an effective edge and they know that edge is often in the mental/emotional arena.

I have played with and against hundreds of quality athletes and every one of them, regardless of how high they have risen in their sport, will tell you that they can "do better still." I've never seen an exception to that. It applies to Olympic athletes as well as to the most highly skilled professional athletes around the world. Furthermore, they all agree that the main barrier to this better performance is the "mental part of the game." Their bodies are highly conditioned and their physical skills are second to none. Thus the difference between a superb day and a so-so one does not lie within their bodies. It resides between their ears. This is fertile territory for a skilled EFT'er.

Experienced golfers, for example, know how to hit every shot perfectly. Their bodies have done it many times. They've hit perfect drives, perfect approach shots, perfect 15-foot putts, and so on. However, despite all their practice and training, golfers don't always shoot perfect rounds. They repeatedly fall below their optimum scores. They play a round of golf and hit a blend of both "perfect shots" and "not-so-perfect" shots and almost invariably end up scoring within their *comfort zone.*

The *comfort zone* is a critical concept within all performance pursuits. This is the mental place where an athlete subconsciously believes he or she "belongs." It is what keeps performance at its current level and, without properly addressing it, any improvements a coach or trainer might develop for an athlete (or musician or actor, etc.) are not likely to be lasting.

Like a thermostat that keeps a room within a comfortable temperature range, our performance fluctuates within certain comfort zones. The comfort zone for golfers, for example, is reflected in their scores. Ask golfers what they shoot and they will answer with something like "the mid 80s" or "the high 70s". This is their comfort zone. It is where they "belong"…even though they will tell you that they can do much better.

Interestingly, improving a specific part of a golfer's game (like putting) will not likely bring about an improved overall score. That's because other parts of the golfer's game will suffer in a manner that will allow the comfort zone (e.g., the mid-80's) to be maintained. Even if golfers have a good day or a bad day and shoot out of their comfort zone, they will, on subsequent rounds shoot once again where they "belong."

To properly enhance one's performance, two factors should be addressed.

1. You must move the comfort zone to better levels, and

2. You must address the specific impediments to performance that need improvement. These sometimes require the proficient EFT'er to address the causative *specific events* in the client's life.

Let's take these two items one at a time.

Adjusting the Comfort Zone

Here are some useful Setup Phrases to help you move beyond your present comfort zone. Please note that they all include a statement of the new level of performance.

This is important in order to move mentally into a new vision of yourself. Feel free to adjust these phrases as needed.

> *Even though I'm uncomfortable shooting in the high 70s and may think I don't belong there, I deeply and completely accept myself.*

> *Even though my free-throw percentage has never been above 80 percent...*

> *Even though I think I am capable of being an A student in math but have never been above a B yet...*

> *Even though the violin doesn't dance in my hands like it does in my dreams...*

> *Even though I have yet to earn $200,000 per year...*

> *Even though, as a speaker, I feel uptight and have yet to have fun with my audience...*

> *Even though I just don't feel attractive and don't have the same outgoing charisma as [pick a role model]...*

> *Even though I go "gulp" instead of flowing freely when I try to sing that high note in [name a song]...*

> *Even though writer's block seems to be always with me instead of ideas flowing out of me like a fountain...*

These go on endlessly and, of course, you must customize these approaches to fit. The idea is to move to a new mental image of yourself in which you see yourself as "belonging" at this new level. Remember, most performers and athletes already believe they have the ability and many of them have already performed at these higher levels, if only briefly. For the most part, they are quite capable of performing beyond their current self-imposed thresholds.

Truly skilled EFT artists do a thorough job with their clients' comfort zones. They dig for the *specific events* underlying their clients' less-than-optimum performance levels and use EFT to obliterate these barriers.

Specific Impediments to Performance

Athletes and performers, like everyone else, are loaded with extraneous bits of self-talk that limit their performance. They pick up thoughts, notions, and attitudes on their journey through life that, once exposed, qualify as first-class comedies.

Let me give you a personal example.

In high school I was a so-so basketball player. My only talent was my ability to jump like a kangaroo and gather rebounds. A rebound is when I get the ball after someone else has missed a shot. As a result I played center for our basketball team, a position normally given to the team's tallest player, someone five or six inches taller than me.

Upon getting a rebound I usually landed within five feet of the basket and often closer. Accordingly, you might think I was the team's leading scorer. After all, my shooting opportunities would have been from short range. But, alas, I only averaged two or three points per game because *I rarely took a shot.* Instead, I passed the ball out to one of the "shooters" on our team. If you think that's silly, you're right. Nonetheless, that's what I did repeatedly.

Why? Because I had developed the self-talk in my head that rebounders are rebounders and that's it. Rebounders are not shooters. This is even more ridiculous when you consider the fact that I had the necessary hand-eye coordination to hit a speeding, curving baseball out of the park and had done so on many occasions. But somehow I had the belief that, because I was a rebounder, I was unable to put a ball into an oversized hoop from a mere five feet away. I can't recall any specific event that gave me this idea, but I suspect I heard a coach or TV announcer comment about a player who was a poor shot because he was such a good rebounder, or some similar opinion was delivered by a person I perceived as expert or authority figure.

Then there was the part of me that was convinced that because I had small hands, I could never dribble a basketball well. The people I perceived as good dribblers were those who could palm the basketball, that is, literally hold it upside down with one hand. There was no way I could do that because my hands were just too small. Therefore, in my mind, I couldn't dribble. Even if I had an open court in front of me with plenty of room to maneuver, I always threw the ball to one of the "dribblers" on our team.

It pains me to look back at my basketball career and see someone who could have been the team's highest scorer throw every opportunity away. Consider that (1) I could out-jump anyone on the team, (2) I grabbed at least a third of the rebounds, (3) I usually landed just a few feet from the basket, (4) the basket was a huge target, practically impossible to miss, and (5) I didn't even try to score. I just threw the ball away. How silly!

In retrospect, I can name many more "comedies" that insidiously eroded my ultimate performance, including my refusal to bat both left- and right-handed in baseball. I had the ability to do this and it would have clearly escalated my batting average. However, I never did it because I was afraid people would see me as a show-off.

I remember in sixth grade hitting left-handed in a softball game, and the ball dribbled past first base. It wasn't much of a hit, but a teacher who was watching exclaimed, "That's the sign of a gifted athlete!" Now, why didn't I pay attention to that response instead of worrying about whether people would think I was conceited?

Dumb...really dumb.

But I can assure you that all performers, regardless of their caliber, carry around dozens of these dandy little dumbos and they aren't even aware they have them. Why? Because they have become routine beliefs and no one has ever helped bring them to the surface so they can be EFT'd out of existence. They have just been buried within and neither the performers nor their coaches, trainers, spouses, or anyone else, has any clue about their existence. Yet these specific impediments to performance serve as unnecessary lids and are monumentally expensive.

It would be great if I could give you a nice clean list of all of these specific impediments to performance, together with a neat and precise recipe for handling each of them.

Alas, a list of these endless comedies would stretch from here to the middle of the Cosmos.

However, with a little creativity and detective work you can soon uncover these hidden thieves. Here are some guidelines.

1. Often there is a disguised "penalty" for performing at one's maximum. Perhaps one thinks that outperforming one's father, mother, brother, or sister will result in a loss of their love. Or maybe someone who achieves that new level will be expected to maintain it (which you might erroneously think will require too much effort). There are many potential penalties. Dig for them. You will often uncover treasure chests filled with ripe issues that need resolution.

2. Sometimes there is a limiting emotional response to a specific competitor, auditorium, academic subject, golf course, etc. I recall many times when a certain pitcher or golf hole or football stadium was "bigger than me." Something about the circumstances "had my number." The resulting self-doubts, of course, affected my play.

3. Many performers focus on what they do well and let slide other aspects of their performance that "aren't as important." However, mastering those other "little things" adds measurably to the overall performance.

Along with the above guidelines I also suggest asking questions like the following:

What does that circumstance or competitor remind you of?

What does your coach or trainer wish you could do?

What prevents you from improving to the next level?

If there was a subconscious penalty for performing even better, what might it be?

Who is better than you and why?

What aspects of your performance have you let slide and why?

What part of your dreams do you consider out of reach or impossible?

When do you have self-doubts? What are they?

What part of your performance do you dislike?

What aspect of your performance are you required to do that you don't like?

Performance issues are mirrors for all those "issues within" that beg for resolution. Quality detective work will almost always find the *specific past events* that limit your own or your client's current performance. Once they're found, EFT is highly likely to collapse them. The result, of course, is a new level of Emotional Freedom that manifests as better scores, better grades, better acting, better writing…and happier people.

Sports Performance and Tail-enders

When you set an ambitious new goal for yourself, listen to what happens on the inside. When you declare a reality that is not currently true, your conflicting issues will often present some opposition, also known as negative self-talk or tail-enders. You might hear something like, *"Sure, when pigs fly." "You know that's impossible." "Forget it." "Why bother?" "Everyone knows I'm just not that good."*

Or take a look at the tail-enders that kept me from excelling. *"I'm a rebounder, and rebounders don't shoot." "If I hit both ways, people will say I'm showing off." "I never win in this ballpark." "The opposition is too good." "My hands are too small."*

Unaddressed, tail-enders have the power to sabotage any goal you try to achieve. On the bright side, tail-enders also point directly to issues you can disarm with EFT, thus removing their power.

Once you identify a specific event that may be contributing to your sports performance problem, you can simply tap the points while telling the story of the event until its emotional intensity is gone. To be more effective, you can identify which emotions you felt during the event and address them individually. For example:

Even though I was humiliated when I made that error and the coach yelled at me, I deeply and completely accept myself.

While tapping the EFT points, use *"this humiliation"* as your Reminder Phrase. Once the emotional intensity for *humiliation* is released, substitute *anger, hopelessness,* or any other feeling that you experienced and address it next.

I consider affirmations and positive goal statements powerful tools in our search for core issues. Pay attention to the part of you that feels uncomfortable when you call yourself a success. Think about where the negative self-talk comes from and see if you can follow it to a specific event. Sometimes the specific event happened recently and sometimes it goes all the way back to childhood. As soon as you find it, tap on it until it's just an old memory, nothing more.

The Personal Peace Procedure, which I described at the end of Chapter One, is an excellent tool for uncovering important past events. Start by listing all the unpleasant, unhappy, disappointing, or frustrating things that have ever happened to you in your sport. Give each event a short title, like a book or movie. Even if you only work on one per day, reducing all that emotional intensity will free your mind for more productive activities, such as reaching your most ambitious goals.

Adapting EFT's Setup Phrase for Sports Performance

An easy way to get started with EFT for improved sports performance is to zero in on a specific problem. What's interfering with your success in scoring points, moving a certain way, running faster, jumping higher, being more flexible, staying focused, or maintaining your stamina?

Start with the basic Setup Phrase as described in Chapter One, which says:

Even though _____, *I deeply and completely accept myself.*

Let's say you're a basketball player, and you just can't score. You could say:

> *Even though I keep missing the basket, I deeply and completely accept myself.*

Now that you have defined the problem, tapping on it may help you feel more relaxed, less anxious, less self-conscious, or less distracted, any of which can improve your performance.

If you define the emotions you feel after missing yet another shot, you can incorporate them into your Setup Phrase. For example:

> *Even though I die of embarrassment every time I miss the basket, I deeply and completely accept myself.*

You can also address individual aspects of the problem, such as:

> *Even though the noise of the crowd really distracts me, I deeply and completely accept myself.*

> *Even though the stiffness in my shoulder interferes with my range of motion, I deeply and completely accept myself, and my body is strong and flexible.*

> *Even though everyone is watching me, and I feel self-conscious, I deeply and completely accept myself.*

You could try a Setup Phrase that helps you move out of your comfort zone. For example:

> *Even though I haven't quite gotten used to relaxing and letting the shots just flow, I deeply and completely accept myself.*

> *Even though it's hard for me to imagine scoring 20 points a game…*

Even though I can see that the basket is an enormous target and it's actually hard to miss...

Even though I have trouble thinking of myself being one of the team's best players, and I'm not sure I belong there...

All of these approaches can help—and one of them might be exactly what you need to leave your scoring problems behind. But if you don't achieve the results you want right away, play detective and look for a past event that is somehow connected to this present problem. As mentioned earlier, an excellent question to ask yourself is:

What does this remind me of?

You may immediately flash back to a game years ago when you missed a shot and someone said something that has interfered with your play ever since. Or maybe you were taller than the rest of the kids and felt self-conscious, a feeling that carried over onto the basketball court. Or maybe your relationship with your girlfriend has been on the rocks and your self-confidence has taken a hit as a result. Or your older brother played for the same team and the thought of out-performing him makes you a little uncomfortable. Or the player you're competing against reminds you of your father or a kid in eighth grade who beat up on you and you feel intimidated. Whatever it might be, let your mind drift until you're back in an event that still carries an emotional charge.

Before tapping, measure your discomfort on the 0-to-10 intensity scale and see how upset you can feel about it now. Remember, this is the *Emotional* Freedom

Techniques, the key word being *Emotion*. Then place the event in a Setup Phrase.

Even though I missed that key shot in the playoffs last year and still feel embarrassed and humiliated because the coach blamed me for losing the game, I deeply and completely accept myself.

Tap through the sequence of EFT points, saying a Reminder Phrase out loud or to yourself at each point, such as *"lost the game," "missed the shot," "embarrassed,"* or *"all my fault."* You can use the same or different Reminder Phrases at each point.

At the end of the sequence, measure the emotional intensity you feel now.

If you feel better but still have some discomfort as you recall the event, tap on your Karate Chop point while saying a new Setup Phrase:

Even though I still have some of this missed shot discomfort, I deeply and completely accept myself.

This time your Reminder Phrase includes the word "remaining," as in *"this remaining missed shot," "remaining embarrassment,"* or *"remaining all my fault."*

Then test your results. When the event no longer holds any emotional charge and thinking about it leaves you feeling relaxed and neutral, try watching a mental movie of the event from start to finish. If that feels comfortable, tell the story out loud to yourself or to a friend. When you can do that without feeling any of the anxiety, tension, or distress that this memory triggered in the past, you have successfully neutralized its emotional charge.

Follow the same strategy with every other aspect or scenario that makes an appearance. For example:

Even though I felt self-conscious about my height all through junior high school and I still get embarrassed when people stare at me, I deeply and completely accept myself. Even though I have always felt uncomfortable standing all by myself at the free throw line, I deeply and completely accept myself, and I play with confidence even with all those people watching.

Even though the coach reminds me of my dad when he criticizes my jump shot and I feel as though I'm still 10 years old and can't do anything right, I deeply and completely accept myself. I know my dad was just frustrated about life and probably so is my coach.

Even though I can't believe Debbie would stand me up like she did Friday night, how could she do that, I deeply and completely accept myself. Even though I'll never understand women, they are just one big mystery to me, I deeply and completely accept myself.

Even though I'm playing almost as well as my brother did, and that makes me uncomfortable, I deeply and completely accept myself. My brother's an adult now. He had his time on the team and now I have mine.

Even though the player I'm competing against reminds me of that kid in sixth grade who stole my lunch money and so I'm a little afraid of him, I deeply and completely accept myself.

A Note about Chronic Injuries

As people in all walks of life have discovered, EFT can be a terrific first-aid treatment. We've received hundreds of reports documenting its use to relieve pain, speed healing, improve range of motion, reduce swelling, prevent bruising, and help the body recover from sprains, muscle pulls, trauma injuries, cuts, abrasions, broken bones, and other mishaps.

You'll find impressive reports from physical therapists and athletes, both here in this book and on our website, describing results that took just a few minutes.

But whenever someone has a chronic problem, such as a sprain or injury that never really goes away, I recommend using the same detective work described above.

Excessive stress or tension always shows up in our muscles. The key question is, what caused it? Maybe you stored a disagreement you had with your wife in your left shoulder. Maybe a friend or relative is the reason behind your knee pain. Sports psychologists seldom factor these causes into their treatments, but EFT practitioners do it all the time.

Whenever a problem doesn't seem to respond to EFT or never completely goes away, look for specific events that may be factors. If you keep this simple strategy in the front of your mind, you'll never be at a loss for effective Setup Phrases, no matter what the problem or challenge.

* * *

Raul Vergini, M.D., who lives in Italy, used EFT with positive self-talk to help a competitive motorcycle rider with his self-confidence. This type of self-confidence building has a wide number of uses. Although there is often more EFT work to do to bring out one's full potential, as described previously, this procedure is valuable just before any sports, acting, or music performance. It's also indispensable for the student before taking a test, for the speaker before that all-important speech, for the fumbling teenager about to go on his or her first date, or for human pursuits of almost any kind.

Dr. Vergini uses a variation of the 0-to-10 intensity scale when he asks the motorcyclist to measure the truth of a damaging self-talk statement. This useful approach is helpful on most issues. I often give people a belief statement relating to their overall issue, such as, *"I'm really angry at the world,"* or, *"My ex-husband was born evil."* I then ask them to repeat it and tell me how true it feels on the 0-to-10 scale. As the session unfolds, this belief statement usually loses its intensity, sounding and feeling less and less true.

EFT for Improved Self-confidence

by Raul Vergini, M.D.

Today I worked with a motorcycle rider. He is German but speaks Italian rather well, and I discovered that he ended in fifth place at the last world championship for 125cc motorcycles.

Talking with him I discovered that he has a problem mainly with two circuits, France and Brazil.

He has always raced poorly in both of them, never achieving better than eighth place in either circuit in the last five years.

As he didn't have any particular emotional feeling about this on the 0-to-10 discomfort scale, I used the same scale to have him measure his beliefs about his performance. I asked how true the statement *"I never can go better than eighth in the France and Rio circuits"* felt. He answered, "Nine." Very true.

After the first round of *"Even though I never can go better than eighth,"* his belief in it went from 9 to 7. We persisted by changing some of the wording to include other possible aspects and it went to 5, then 3, then 2.

Then — and this is important to recognize — I realized that when he was at a 2 he was actually giving me the rating for *"I cannot win in France or Brazil."*

So I told him, "Wait a minute, we are shifting to another statement now. We started with a 9 regarding the *'eighth position'* phrase, but now we are at 2 with the *'I cannot win'* phrase. It's a completely different thing! How intense now is the old 'eighth place' belief?" He said, "Oh, it went down to zero some time ago!" We laughed and quickly zeroed in on *"I cannot win in France and Brazil,"* which, of course, had already almost disappeared.

✻ ✻ ✻

EFT can generate impressive benefits for every sport from soccer to platform diving to anything else. This is because the principles are the same regardless of the activity. To emphasize this, Guillermo Penia from Spain lists his accomplishments using EFT for nautical sports. Guillermo tapped physically before his race, then he tapped mentally during the race itself, and he broke the event's overall record.

Want to be a Champion?

by Guillermo Penia

I will present the results I have obtained using EFT in sports over the last two years. Parallel to my activities in EFT, I teach Nautical Sports. In the spring of 2006, I decided to test the results of EFT in competitions. I decided to train to attempt to break Spanish Record in Kite Boarding in Long Distance Speed. I used EFT on everything: physical factors, self-esteem, motivation, and even to get a sponsor so I could dedicate myself fully to the project.

Finally on August 26 of the same year, I sailed 46 nautical miles with an average speed of 22.6 knots (26.0 mph or 41.8 kph). Not only did I break the Spanish Record, I won and still hold the World Record. What surprised me most was that everything was so easy.

A few months later I found myself thinking, "I have been practicing kiteboard for many years and the physical effort in it is minimal because it is the wind that does the work." So I decided to do something different and unknown to me. I found out about SUP (Stand Up Paddle Surf) and decided to give it a try. In this sport in order to move forward, it is necessary to paddle so you have to make continuous physical effort.

I set as my goal participating in the August 2008 SUP International Championship "nine nautical miles" held in Santa Pola, Spain.

In order to qualify for the Championship, I had to become one of the top-ranking competitors in Spain. To achieve this I had to participate in short-distance races, called Open Races. I became the Spanish runner-up in this modality.

In the weeks before the Championship, the aspects to be treated with EFT were so many that my wife, Ilka, offered to be my motivating coach.

For the International Championship I did tapping before the race and also mentally while racing, and I finished first with more than two minutes advantage over the runner-up, breaking the nine-mile overall record.

I say all this not to brag about myself or my successes but to emphasize the excellent results of applying EFT to oneself, to show the great potential of EFT and the significant changes that can happen in one's life, all of which are applicable to every single aspect of it and serve to broaden your horizons to wherever you set the limits.

My physical constitution is average. I won the SUP International Championship at 49 years of age to the amazement of the press and fellow sportsmen.

Thanks to Gary and to everyone else involved in help-ing expand the EFT horizons!

※ ※ ※

This next report is an excellent demonstration of EFT in practice from Alvaro Munoz of Colombia. Its focus is a Japanese martial art, but the same approach can work for any sport in which our impatience, anxiety, apprehen-sion, discouragement, worry, mental criticisms, and other negative emotions get in the way.

EFT and Aikido

by Alvaro Munoz

Aikido is a Japanese martial art in which one redirects the attacker´s energy and returns it to him or her. Although I am a Karate black belt and have some experience in martial arts, I must confess that Aikido is a world apart. Every technique I used in order to learn Karate failed when learning Aikido. I practiced and practiced and practiced for years, but my performance wouldn't go above a certain level, and then it suddenly started to slow down. So did my enthusiasm. I felt disappointed, tired, frustrated, and even anxious. I considered surrendering but, know-ing it would only make me feel guilty, decided to keep practicing. However, I was attending the dojo more as a habit than anything else and soon found myself mak-ing excuses to avoid the practice…until I tried EFT.

First of all, I checked all the limiting beliefs about my practicing Aikido and tapped for them:

Even though Aikido is so hard to learn, I deeply and completely accept myself.

Even though I can't relax during the practice...

Even though I have no time to practice...

Then I tapped for my feelings when practicing:

Even though I feel anxious, I deeply and completely accept myself.

Even though I want my hakama (kind of black belt degree)...

Even though I want to understand this discipline...

Even though I feel so stressed when my teacher approaches...

Even though newer mates are doing better than I am...

Even though I try and I try and I try...

Even though my shoulders are so stressed during the practice...

Even though I don't understand Aikido...

Even though I am competing with myself...

Even though I am putting so much pressure on myself...

Even though I am not enjoying this...

Finally I realized that the emotion that kept me from improving was my anxiety, so I tapped again with the following Setup Phrases:

*Even though I am so anxious about being a master,
I deeply and completely accept myself.*

*Even though I want to be a master <u>now</u>, I have the
power to remain relaxed, centered, and calm.*

*Even though I want to do everything right the first
time, I am always in my territory (myself).*

*Even though I want to be fast, I have the power to
remain relaxed, centered, and calm.*

I did this recently for about an hour. I tapped on
everything coming to my mind about Aikido and anxiety. Today, before my practice, I did four or five more
rounds, just in case…and guess what.

My practice was so cool! I was completely
relaxed, my shoulders didn't disturb my posture, my
arms were moving freely, and even when I saw my
sensei (teacher) coming, I didn't felt that weird sense
of being observed and judged. Rather, I performed
with the intention that as she corrected me, I would
feel confident and totally enjoy the practice.

I also noticed that after the anxiety-tapping session, my body feels much more relaxed when driving.
I will keep tapping on everything that arises as well as
before every practice.

❋ ❋ ❋

What might happen if you consistently used EFT
to collapse your emotional "limits"? Would a "new you"
arise? Read this article by Cathie van Rooyen from South
Africa for a clue about the new vistas that may await you.

Like many runners who use EFT, Cathie taps on her finger points, which are described in Appendix A.

EFT Turned Me into a Marathon Runner

by Cathie van Rooyen

I have been practicing EFT for many years and have discovered an unusual side effect. It turned me into a marathon runner. Now, I have never consciously tapped on turning myself into an athlete because I had a love affair with my couch. I had no interest whatsoever in running around my neighborhood block, never mind from city to city. Three years later while running a 50-kilometer (31-mile) road race, it struck me that it might just be a side effect of using EFT. I have tapped on self-esteem issues, self-confidence issues, procrastination, and other emotional issues, but not once did I tap on "I want to be a runner."

I have now run distances which make my mind boggle, and last year I attempted our ultra road race of 88 kilometers (55 miles). This year I am going to do it again. I have tapped on various issues which I now experience as a runner, while faced with distance and heat and blisters. But overall, I have found myself at the starting line time and time again, with no nervousness, no self-doubt, only excitement. The challenge doesn't scare me, and I have given up the old internal dialogue of, "Who do you think you are, trying to run this?"

While running, I have tapped on my fingers for things like:

Even though I have these heavy legs, I deeply and completely accept myself.

Even though it's so far...

Even though my chest feels tight...

Even though there are blisters on my toes...

Even though I am not an athlete...

Even though I never finish anything...

Even though I am not fast enough...

Even though I am too overweight...

Even though I am too old...

Even though I am not a runner...

All of these issues no longer bother me. I am excited by the prospect of seeing my world on foot. I enjoy the sights and sounds of all the different types of runners on the road. I am enjoying the challenge of willing my body to the finish line. I have new pride in my body, huge respect for my legs, my feet, my body. All of this I attribute to EFT. I now warn my clients, who look rather alarmed when I joke about this particular side effect! Thank you, Gary, and warn your clients, too!

❊ ❊ ❊

Dawn Norton used EFT to help both of her sons with their tennis performance. But performance was not the only benefit. Here's a success story in more ways than one.

Success on the Tennis Court

by Dawn Norton

Last fall I started studying EFT seriously. I have been so thrilled with the improvements it has made in emotional, physical, and achievement areas of my life. We have had much success in our family with it.

Even though my children have heard multiple stories and we have had our own successes, there still tends to be a reluctance in some of them, and I couldn't wait to try it with them with their sports.

They went through basketball season without taking advantage of EFT. But when tennis started, my oldest came and asked me to help him. So, as the season started, we sat down for a "session" and he told me all the things he felt needed improvement. His footwork. Playing at the net. His serve. And tossing the ball up and getting it just right before he hit it. We spent close to an hour tapping for these and other problems:

Even though I have a hard time approaching the net, I deeply and completely accept myself.

Even though my footwork stinks…

Even though I have this toss problem…

Even though my serve needs improving…

I am happy to report that he feels much better about his abilities, he appears to be playing better, and he has been ranked number one or two the whole season at our school. He did not come near that last year.

Enter son #2. When he came home from tennis workouts in which everyone plays each other and they are ranked, he told me he had played a particularly difficult friend (personality, not skill) and that he decided he was going to tap about it. He said he did not want to be embarrassed by tapping all over, so he only tapped on his Karate Chop point. The only Setup he shared with me was:

Even though I don't want to lose to _____, I deeply and completely accept myself.

And what a difference it made! My son can be a little volatile at times, but he reported that he did not get angry, throw his racket, smash balls over the fence, or swear in his mind. Further, even though he lost to this friend, he was able to shake his hand and tell him it was a good game.

Instead of the usual complaints and anger I hear from him about frustrating game situations, I heard a maturing young man tell me how he conquered his frustrations with just a little bit of tapping on one EFT point! Win or lose, this comes through as a great success in my book.

❊ ❊ ❊

In this next report, pay particular attention to how Marla Tabaka listens to her client and digs out important core issues. Whenever Mark's intensity level shot back up after coming down, he was focusing on a different aspect, a different facet of the problem. By addressing each aspect as a new or separate issue, Maria demonstrates the art of delivery that makes EFT both fast and effective. Notice too how she incorporates the physical symptoms that reflected his stress and anxiety. These symptoms disappeared when the emotional blocks interfering with his sports performance were removed.

EFT Secures College Football Scholarship

by Marla Tabaka

This summer I was contacted by the father of a 17-year-old high school place kicker. His son, "Mark," had a sudden onset of issues around performing under pressure at college camps. Mark's athletic abilities are outstanding and he has no problem achieving peak performance levels in practice and in most games. However, after a lifetime of striving toward college-level play, Mark's performance abilities were mediocre at best during camp competitions where high school level football players vie for the coveted invitation to join high-ranking schools across the nation.

Simply by imagining himself performing at an upcoming camp, Mark's discomfort level rose to a 9. The intensity level was measured not only by an emotional fear-of-failure response, but tingling in his legs and heaviness in his chest. He also bounced his foot excessively and I noticed that Mark's ears turned red whenever we talked about an upcoming competition.

In an attempt to make Mark feel more comfortable during our first session, we worked on the tingling and tightness, but he did not show much improvement because so many negative scenarios were dancing in his head. So we moved on to those. Since he'd never performed badly before, Mark had no negative memories contributing to his fears.

After about an hour of processing and opening the various doors with EFT, Mark realized that the camps have exposed him to other players who are as good as or better than he is. In his limited experience, Mark had never encountered a peer with equal abilities and he was not prepared for this realization. He began to question whether he deserved a scholarship award and whether the coaches would even notice him.

Beginning with an intensity level of 9 on the 0-to-10 scale for the tingling, heaviness, and very reddened ears, we began our Setup with:

Even though I have more competition than I've ever bargained for—and that's shocking and scary—I deeply and completely accept myself.

Even though I have this fear of the unexpected competition...

Even though I really don't like that I'm not number one anymore...

A couple of rounds only brought the level of intensity down to 8 in his fear and 7 for the tingling and heaviness. So we moved on to:

Even though I don't deserve this scholarship as much as the others do, and I feel frustrated about that…

After one round of tapping, his intensity came down to a 4. It jogged Mark's memories of feeling cocky and overly confident in the beginning of his junior year, when he didn't work as hard as he now feels he should have.

Even though my ego got in the way and I got lazy about my goals and now I feel frustrated and angry with myself for that…

After one round of tapping on that, his level of intensity shot up to a 9 out of 10 again. Why? Because now Mark felt a ton of guilt about letting down his teammates and his parents.

Even though I let everyone down, including myself, and I really let that ego get in the way, and now I have this guilt that feels like a ton of bricks sitting on my chest and legs…

After two rounds of tapping on "this frustration and guilt," we used a new Setup with an overall level of intensity of 5:

Even though I have this ton of guilt-bricks on my chest and legs, I choose to forgive the 16-year-old in me who had a cocky ego and allow my now mature and driven side to surface freely with confidence and joy.

I forgive that 16-year-old in me and relieve myself of this burden of guilt. After all, I was only 16 and now my ego is safely tucked away.

I now remove these bricks of guilt, feeling my breath grow deeper and deeper as each brick is lifted.

We tapped for a full round and Mark's color returned to normal and his breathing was deep and relaxed. His level of intensity was zero out of 10 with no tingling and no heaviness. Now he felt deserving, relaxed, and confident.

After performing flawlessly at the next camp (he tapped on his nervousness before going on the field), Mark was offered a scholarship to his second-choice college. He's keeping his fingers crossed for number one, but has gained the confidence to go in as a "walk on" and work toward some scholarship money at his number-one choice school.

Mark continues to come to EFT coaching sessions twice a month because he feels so at peace after working on his goals. The sessions have not only had an impact on Mark's athletic goals but his spiritual awareness as well.

❖ ❖ ❖

As a novice who learned to ski at age 50, New York resident Lillian Fimbres took a tumble that made one particular trail too scary to contemplate. She avoided it for three years. Then she learned EFT and that made all the difference.

Skiing with EFT

by Lillian Fimbres

I started skiing when I was 50, compared to most skiers who start when they're right out of the crib. That's an exaggeration—they at least can stand. When you grow up skiing, you have a chance to deal with the fear factor gradually. The movements come with less resistance and the experience is more fluid and natural, or so it seems to me. I on the other hand had acquired 50 years worth of fear in all its shapes and forms, which can subconsciously cancel out any confidence or athletic ability I might think I have for such a thing as learning to ski. The fears include things like skiing too fast and out of control, not being able to stop, crashing into trees, people, and small children, skiing off the trail into the snowy wooded abyss, falling off the lift, breaking bones, hips, wrists, fingers, or head, and the worst fear for skiers, tearing the anterior cruciate ligament, or ACL. Yet, despite my bruised, battered, and twisted body, I was determined to ski better each time I went up the lift. I rapidly improved with instruction and had the basics more or less under my belt in the first two years. What I didn't have was experience or common sense.

There was one trail in particular that I avoided for three years. It was a black diamond trail called Belleayre Run that you could see going up on the lift to the top of the mountain. Trails are categorized by color. For instance, black diamond trails are for the more advanced skier. Blue trails are usually groomed and considered to be intermediate trails for the safe recreational skier. The green trails are the bunny slopes where most skiers get their first bruises and sprains. I decided that this was the day that I would graduate from the intermediate to the more advanced trails. I had always wanted to ski Belleayre Run. It looked so inviting from the chairlift and it wasn't particularly crowded that day at the resort. I could take my time getting down and not feel rushed. It seemed like the next natural step for me to advance my skills. The snow looked good, the sun was out, skiers and snowboarders seemed to be having an easy time coming down. The time was now or never. Despite my fears and my apprehension, today was the day I would ski down Belleayre Run with my experienced skiing buddy, Dolores, keeping an eye on me.

For some reason which may not be important to the story, Dolores and I didn't ride up together. The plan was we were going to meet at the top of Belleayre Run. The first one there would wait for the other. That was the first mistake I made because it takes about 12 minutes from the base to summit on that old chairlift. It's so slow. One of the first commandments a beginner skier should obey is never ever stop and wait at the top a steep trail by oneself for 12 minutes. The trail only gets steeper and icier with each passing second, and skiers whizzing past me laughing and cajoling made it even worse on my nerves. How could they be yukking it up, having all that fun when my body was getting tenser and my boots were starting to kill me? I was changing my mind about this, but it was too late to ski down the easy way. I was committed. No turning back unless I wanted to inch my way back up the hill to the bunny slopes with my tail between my legs.

Dolores arrived and I pushed off with her as my 911 emergency backup. Sure enough, into my very first turn I attempted to ski back up the hill, probably looking for my mommy. This caused me to fall and I wound up lying upside down at the very top of the trail. It's one thing to fall and be in a predicament near the bottom of the trail where you don't have too far to slide until the terrain flattens out, but when you're upside down at the top, it's a whole different story. So many more bad things can still happen. Every time I tried to turn my body around so my skis faced downhill instead up in the air I would start sliding downhill backwards. Luckily, my 911 came to my rescue and with a few careful pole plants I got turned around. My nerves were shattered by the time I skied down.

I became quite a good skier during the next three years, but I avoided my nemesis. I've skied steeper trails then Belleayre Run under worse conditions, yet I made every excuse not to ski it: it's too crowded, the snow is skied off, they didn't groom it, it's too icy, too soft, too wet, there's too much crud, it's too late in the day, too early in the day, too foggy, too overcast, the lighting is too flat, visibility is poor, the sun's not out, it's too windy, I'm tired, I'll go next time when I have the legs.

Then I learned EFT. I had a few more trips lined up for spring skiing, and I was excited to see if it would really help me conquer my old pal, Belleayre Run. I tapped like a crazy women going up the chairlift and used the restraining bar to tap my Karate Chop point against. Luckily I rode the chairlift up by myself so I could tap away with great abandon.

Even though I'm scared to death, I deeply and completely accept myself.

Even though this trail spooked me, I'm a really good skier.

Even though I'm afraid to ski Belleayre Run, I know I have the skills to come down the mountain in one piece.

Even though I'm nervous, I know I'll be amazed as to how easy this trail is because I know how to ski.

Then I tapped on my reminder points through my gloves, my helmet, my goggles, and my ski jacket. *This fear, this fear. I'm a good skier. This is going to be so much fun. I know how to control my speed. I can do this. I can ski relaxed and be in control. This fear, this fear. Even if I fall it won't be a big deal.*

And so on.

I had such a big smile on my face skiing down the mountain. Everything came together and I felt grounded and playful on my skis. I was ecstatic when

I stopped at the bottom of the trail and looked back up the mountain. That kind of elation doesn't leave you. For a skier it becomes fuel for the next challenge. In skiing when you fall, wipe out, and crash so badly that skis and poles go flying in one direction while goggles, gloves, and hat take off in another, it's called a yard sale. EFT has made a huge difference in my skiing. It has helped me get down the mountain without having so many yard sales!

※ ※ ※

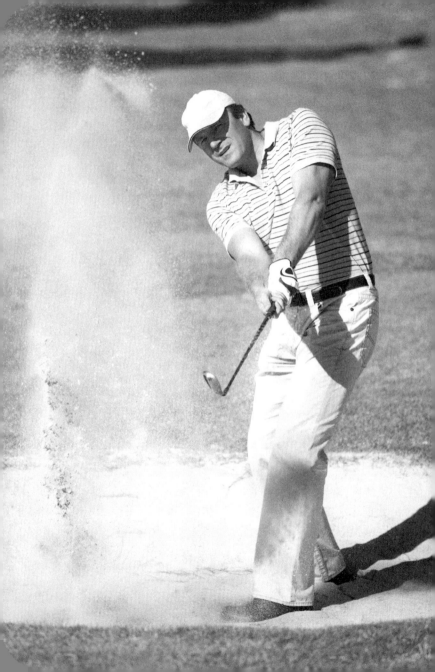

3

EFT Sports Statistics

Using EFT to enhance sports performance not only provides results that the eyes can clearly see, but it also produces results that we can easily measure via statistics. Thus we can apply EFT and undeniably demonstrate its effectiveness by pointing to improvements in golf scores, basketball shooting percentages, baseball batting averages, football field goal statistics, and on and on it goes.

Not every sport lends itself to such straightforward statistical proof, however. Exceptions might be the more artistic sports such as synchronized swimming, ballroom dancing, figure skating, diving, or gymnastics. But even in these cases, improved performance can be readily discerned in the eyes of the judges.

In this book's introduction I mentioned a study ("The Effect of Energy Psychology on Athletic Performance: A Randomized Controlled Blind Trial") presented by Dawson Church, Ph.D., at the tenth annual conference of the Association for Comprehensive Energy Psychology, or ACEP, in May 2008. The study showed impressive improvements in the completion of free throws by high-performance basketball players at Oregon State University after they used EFT. The same school's baseball team won two consecutive College Baseball World Series championships after adopting EFT.

Here are some informal studies that confirm EFT's effectiveness.

In 1999, back in the early days of EFT, a pitcher in the Australian Baseball League learned how to use EFT. Pat Ahearne had been drafted by the Detroit Tigers in 1992 and made his major league debut in 1995. By 1998, he was living in Australia, where he played for the Perth Heat.

If you are familiar with baseball statistics you will find Pat's "before and after EFT" statistics very impressive. Pay particular attention to the Earned Run Average, or ERA. This is the main yardstick by which pitchers are measured. The lower, the better. Rarely do you find any pitcher, anywhere, get as low as Pat's 0.87.

Please note in Pat's message that he maintained his improved performance and did so with major improvement in his durability and endurance. As you read this, please think about the professional athletes who tend to wear down at the end of a season. Most of them have to "suck it up" and play with injuries and tired bodies. What is it worth for them to be in top condition during those all-important playoff rounds, including the World Series (baseball), the Super Bowl (football), and the NBA playoffs (basketball)?

In the ten years that followed this 1999 report, Pat Ahearne played baseball around the world. He now runs a summer baseball camp in Florida and is on the staff of the Rod Dedeaux Research and Baseball Institute as a pitching instructor and International Coordinator.

Pitcher of the Year, Thanks to EFT

by Pat Ahearne

As anyone who has competed in athletics can say, the difference between the average athlete and the elite player is much more mental than physical. In an effort to bring my mental preparation for baseball to the same level as my physical preparation, I was introduced to EFT by Steve Wells, a psychologist based in Perth, Australia. Before working with Steve, I was able to perform well in training and some of the time in games, but I wanted to access my best performances more often and in the most pressure-filled situations.

Steve and I worked together using EFT to lessen or eliminate the mental and emotional barriers preventing me from consistently producing my best games as a pitcher. The results were astounding. I had more consistency and better command of my pitches, and I accomplished this in big games with less mental effort. There is clear evidence in the numbers when you compare my 1998-1999 Australian Baseball League season statistics before EFT and after EFT:

	Win-Loss Record	Innings Pitched	Hits Given Up	Earned Runs	Walks Given Up	Strike-outs	Earned Run Ave.
Before EFT	4–2	46	43	17	18	35	33.3
After EFT	3–1	41.3	15	4	7	37	0.87

With EFT, I found the mental edge that raises an athlete from average to elite. I used the techniques to capture the awards for Most Valuable Player (MVP) of the Perth Heat and the Australian Baseball League Pitcher of the Year.

I am so amazed with the effectiveness of EFT that I've made it as important a part of my baseball routine as throwing or running or lifting weights. The title "Emotional Freedom Techniques" certainly does fit.

[*My comment:* Here is an update Pat sent three years later.]

I was looking for an article of mine in New Haven this season and stumbled across my testimonial and follow-up on your site. I just returned from a winter-ball assignment in Venezuela where I got another 40 innings pitched with a 2.05 ERA. Things are progressing well and I am continuing to work over the telephone with Steve Wells.

I also have something to add that might further the worth of the techniques in the area of durability and endurance. I can best illustrate this with a comparison.

My longest season in terms of innings pitched prior to my 1998-1999 season in Perth [when EFT was first used] was 142 innings pitched in '95 for Toledo (AAA Detroit Tigers). After that season I was physically and mentally drained and looked forward to a five-month off-season.

Compare this to the stretch from November 1998 to December 1999 [during which time EFT was applied]. I pitched 87 innings in Perth followed by a combined 170 innings in Bridgeport and New Haven, Connecticut, and finally another 40 innings in Venezuela for a total of 297 innings pitched in a 13-month span. This is over twice the innings pitched —without any sustained rest periods.

Add that to the fact that I feel physically and mentally strong and am confident I will be at my best again when spring training arrives in March on only three months rest from competitive situations.

Also, my Earned Run Average during that 297-inning span was: Perth 2.16, Bridgeport 2.45, New Haven 2.61, and Venezuela 2.05. All those numbers are over a full run better than any season I had in my professional career. That's over a 30-percent improvement. I can't ask for much better results, and they have carried over the course of a long and taxing baseball season.

I just wanted to add that extra bit which is better seen from the end-of-the-season perspective. If there is anything I can do to help you out, don't hesitate to contact me. As Steve has said, I hope to help put EFT in the headlines.

❊ ❊ ❊

Judy Whitcraft of Kansas City, Kansas, uses EFT with her tumbling students and has compiled statistics documenting their impressive improvement. As Judy says, EFT is so easy, even a seven-year-old can use it!

EFT Statistics from a Tumbling Team

by Judy Whitcraft

For 37 years I have owned my own tumbling/dance studio. Tumbling consists of cartwheels, handsprings, and other moves that are performed on a tumbling mat like floor exercise in gymnastics. For over a year I used EFT in the tumbling classes that I teach in the studio as well as for our tumbling team.

Our team competes in three tumbling meets each year. Eighty girls from age 3 to 16 competed this past season with our team.

The first two meets are qualifying meets, and then there is a championship trophy meet where only the winners from the first two meets compete in their age and skill division. My girls have always done extremely well in qualifying for the championship and in bringing home trophies.

This year, on the back of the tumbling meet entry form, I added a release form for parents to sign giving me permission to use EFT with their children in order to enhance peak performance. At the first practice, I demonstrated EFT for flexibility and had the parents tap along with the children. EFT was very well received by most all the girls and parents, and we definitely saw results at the practices.

A few of the Setup Phrases we used included:

Even though my toes weren't pointed, I have great muscles.

Even though my splits are not all the way down, I have a flexible body.

Even though I didn't land my trick, my body knows how to do it.

Even though I don't like to be judged, I choose to have fun anyway.

Even though I am afraid I might mess up and feel bad, I am an awesome kid anyway.

And of course we used EFT for headaches, breathing problems, strained muscles, fear, and general pain.

One practice with an advanced group of 10- to 11-year-olds had an interesting outcome. The girls had to be there for two hours, and after only 45 minutes, they were tired, irritable, acting silly, and wasting everyone's time. I sat them down in a circle, and we all tapped together:

Even though I don't want to be here and my mom is making me stay, I choose to have a great practice.

Even though Judy is being mean and I just want to go home and play, I can have fun anyway.

Even though I don't want to do this, you can't make me, I don't wanna, and I ain't gonna, I'm still an awesome kid.

The change was *miraculous!* For the rest of the practice *all* eight of the girls were energetic, cooperative, worked hard, got a lot accomplished, *and had fun!* Thank you, EFT!

After the Championship tumbling meet in March, as I printed out the list of trophy winners to display on the wall, I kept thinking that the 48 trophies we won were more than we had ever received before. This prompted me to put together statistics to see if this were so. The figures showed we had brought home 28 percent more trophies than the previous year! Then I went back five years and put those statistics together. There were approximately 80 girls on the team each year, so that variable was minimal. When I averaged the five previous years together, we had upgraded that number by 45 percent!

In addition, the places won were higher, with more firsts, seconds, and thirds. When I gave each place a value like at a track meet, scoring 6 team points for first, 5 team points for second, etc., the figures between 2005 and 2006 showed a 30-percent increase. Over the past five-year average, it was a 43-percent increase. So the level of placement was high, along with the number of trophies.

Three of the mothers told me they tapped with their children in the car all the way to the tumbling meet. Other mothers reported stories of improvement at practices at home using EFT. I decided to take a survey of how the girls had used EFT on their own, away from the studio. The results showed that:

- 63 percent tapped the day of the meet.

- 60 percent tapped while practicing at home.

- 63 percent tapped for other issues when away from the studio.

- 47 percent said other members of their family now use EFT.

- 26 percent have taught friends to use EFT.

The girls also used EFT for a variety of issues other than their tumbling skills. And they all reported successful results! Most of the girls are elementary school age! They used EFT for headaches, ear aches, ear blockages, runny noses, toothaches, neck aches, allergies, asthma, riding a bike, endurance running, basketball, softball, swimming, karate, math speed cards, math homework, spelling, achievement test fear, thunderstorms, climbing a tree, and when they are mad at their friends.

Many of my instructors and assistants also reported that they are using EFT on their own and with others.

When children work on a skill, I coach them on what to change during their next turn, and they tap all the way back to line saying, "Kick harder," or, "Arms up on hop." This not only taps it in but it makes them pay attention to the coaching and focus on it. My very favorite is when they do the skill well and I have them tap all the way back to line, saying, "I did good," "I am wonderful," "I am awesome," or, "I did it."

Another favorite is when a child is close to perfecting a new skill, I have everyone focus on that person while tapping on their Karate Chop points, sending positive energy to the performer. It not only gives the child an extra boost but lets the rest of the team contribute to the success of a classmate.

I have many stories about children coming back from a slight injury in a very few minutes. Since I am usually teaching class when that happens, I often send one of the assistants (age 12-15) to tap with the student.

Lately I have been collecting stories about how the girls ages 8 to 14 have used EFT on their own, away from the studio. Many said they used EFT at school to focus and calm down before tests. Many said they had used it for headaches, stomach aches, sprained ankles, etc. Many use it for sports performance in soccer, softball, track, weight lifting, etc. for endurance, precision, and eliminating fear. The age 11–13 group reported using EFT when they were angry at their parents, siblings, and friends.

Nicole, age 10, said she tapped when her kitty got hurt and she was scared its leg was going to have to be cut off. Kylie, age 11, said she tapped at the hospital when she was afraid her grandma was going to die. Quinlynn, age 11, said she always has the flu for three days, but this time she tapped many times during the first day of being sick, and she got over it in *one day!* Trisha, age 14, tapped on her 12-year-old brother when he was "freaking out" in the car when a tornado was a mile behind them on the highway. Tonya, age 14, taps for the tendonitis in her elbow and this keeps the swelling down after softball practice. Kristin, age 14, finally was able to get her contacts lenses in, after eight years of trying! Taylor, age 12, tapped on her friend at the track meet, and her friend set a new school record in the high jump! (And her friend gave credit to "that tapping stuff.") Seven-year-old Anna said she tapped before a soccer game and scored a goal!

Six-year-old Ashley was throwing a fit getting dressed for class because her mother had not brought the leotard she wanted. I asked her mother if she wanted me to tap on her. Definitely she did! I took Ashley to a private area and asked her if I could tap on her. She said OK, so I had her tap while repeating my phrases: *"I don't want to wear this." "It is ugly." "It doesn't fit right." "My mom can't make me wear it." "I'm making her go home and get the other one."* Within two minutes, Ashley was smiling and running out to class with her friends. She was in a great mood the whole class. From meltdown to happy in two minutes!

One day at recital before going onstage, I found a whole group of seven- and eight-year-olds tapping together to smile on stage. They ended up winning second place for the overall class recital smiling award, which is amazing for that age group.

I love that these children are discovering their own power and actually using it to improve their emotional and physical health! I have been very pleased with the receptive attitude in our small community. Of course some roll their eyes and laugh, but the results speak for themselves. My thanks to you for making EFT so easy that even a seven-year-old can use it.

❄ ❄ ❄

Sam Smith from Australia kept accurate data during a rugby kicking contest. The participants took free kicks from various distances and did so both before and after doing EFT. So that the results could be readily assessed, I put Sam's data into tables and calculated the success rates. The improvements are obvious. If you calculate summaries of the "before" and "after" success rates, you end up with an overall improvement of 80.7 percent. Also, the number of "misses that hit the post or bar"— that is, they came very close to succeeding—went from 15 to 163 for an overall improvement of 986.7 percent.

While it's true that part of this improvement could be attributed to "getting better with practice," I spent my formative years heavily involved in highly competitive athletics and, in my experience, only 10 to 20 percent of this change could be attributed to that factor.

Impressive Rugby Kicking Improvement

by Sam Smith

Last weekend I attended a local fundraiser. I find these occasions useful to promote EFT. I give out informational flyers and try to cater the presentation of EFT to the type of event. Usually the spot costs us a donation to the organization of anywhere from $25 to $100, which is well worth it for the exposure.

Because this event took place on sporting fields, I set up a kicking competition using EFT as a "relaxing and focusing" method to aid the kickers and offered prizes as an incentive. The exercise involved taking rugby penalty kicks, using an oval rugby ball. I used rugby because I'm a soccer player and I felt that to kick a rugby ball was more challenging. The ball was placed on a kicking tee and the aim was to get as many over the bar and between the posts as possible.

We used ten different penalty spots. They were all directly in front of the goals and set at the following distances: 20 meters, 25 meters, 30 meters, 35 meters, and 40 meters. (One meter is 39.4 inches, or slightly more than a yard.)

Volunteers of both genders age 12 to 54 years were given a few minutes to warm up then took a total of ten place kicks. They had two kicks per distance. The weather was dry but there was a bit of a breeze from their left. At the end they were asked to state what two things they believed prevented them from scoring better and which could improve their score for the second round of kicking.

The following statements were most common:

I'm not a rugby player. I'm not strong enough. I don't have the proper boots; shoes; kit for this; etc. It's too hard from that distance; from this distance; from this spot. I have no technique. It's been years since I've kicked a ball. I play real football (soccer). The wind was against me.

The wind is too strong. Too many people were watching. I never do well at this type of thing. Well, it's only a bit of fun. I knew I couldn't do it.

I knew I couldn't do it. My aim was off. I was aiming too low. I was aiming too high.

When the volunteers (37 during the course of the day) completed their first rounds, they were shown how to "relax and focus" using EFT Setups on their statements followed by a full shortcut round of tapping with appropriate Reminder Phrases. This was done prior to their second attempt and again whenever they felt it necessary.

Collectively on the first round the results were:

Distance	Attempts	Successes	Percent Successes
20 meters	370	71	19.2%
25 meters	370	118	31.9%
30 meters	370	74	20%
35 meters	370	55	14.9%
40 meters	370	35	9.5%

(Misses that hit the post or bar = 15)

On the second round:

Distance	Attempts	Successes	Percent Successes
20 meters	370	116	31.4%
25 meters	370	179	48.4%
30 meters	370	133	36%
35 meters	370	125	33.8%
40 meters	370	85	23%

(Misses that hit the post or bar = 163)

With more time and attention we could have improved everybody's kicking beyond their wildest imagination, but the time restraints and staffing did not allow me to delve further.

What was evident to those participating and watching was how each individual's second round of penalty kicks came much closer to going over. This was a startling observation for many. This result clearly indicates the power of EFT in this simplest but very important part of just one sport.

* * *

Dawson Church spent a mere 15 minutes doing EFT with a competitive dancer who dramatically improved the height of his kicks. Note the statistics given (one kick improved by 22 percent) and how Dawson introduced the "safety catch" phrase within the EFT Setup statement.

Competitive Dancer Improves Performance
by Dawson Church, Ph.D.

Every athlete strives to break his or her previous best record. Athletes measure their times and numbers, then work hard on the aspects of their performance that impair their ability to do better. Each sport has one or more measures, such as free throws in basketball, goal kicks in soccer, and points in gymnastics. EFT can be used by athletes to improve those metrics, and there are many accounts of athletes quickly seeing huge improvements in performance after applying EFT.

However, when trying to break a physical barrier, it's important to avoid injury. If ligaments and tendons are stretched beyond their limits, they tear, as countless limping athletes can tell you. Trying to exceed their limits, they tear rotator cuffs in their shoulders. They blow out the meniscus cartilages in their knees. They come down with tennis elbow or carpal tunnel syndrome. If an athlete is getting good results with EFT, it's tempting to push harder and take risks at the limit of the envelope of performance. That's why I believe it's important to add a "safety catch" to your Setup Phrase, especially if you're doing rapid or strenuous exercise that gives you scant time to pull back if you reach beyond the limits of safety.

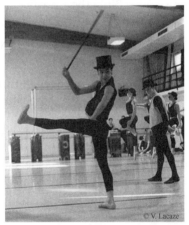

An Athletic Ballet Kick Called a *Battement*

Here's an example of using both a Setup Phrase that stretches you toward a goal and a safety catch that stops you from getting injured. I recently visited a friend's home and talked to her eighteen-year-old son. He's an avid dancer who dances competitively in swing, tango, waltz, and ballet.

He was complaining about his performance limitations in certain ballet moves, so I suggested we try EFT. The two particular moves that were giving him trouble are called a *battement* and a *grande battement.* They both involve kicks straight out front, but with different hip positions, resulting in a higher kick for the grande battement. Think of the Rockettes at Radio City Music Hall doing their high kicks and you'll get the picture.

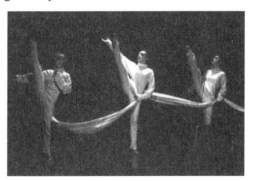

A Chorus Line Performing Grande Battements

I measured his performance on both kicks using marks on the edge of a wall. I had him perform three of his best kicks for both moves, standing with the big toe of his other leg in the same marked spot. He was remarkably consistent, within about a quarter-inch range over all three kicks. I took careful measurements from the floor to within one-quarter inch of his average.

Then we did EFT. His particular challenge is that, while his muscles are strong and his ligaments are very flexible, the muscles of his upper thigh (quadriceps and adductors) contract involuntarily when he performs a kick, limiting the range of travel of his leg.

So our Setup statement was,

Even though the muscles in my upper thigh are tight and interfere with kicking, I deeply and completely accept myself.

Even though they are tight, the muscles of my upper thigh remain relaxed when I kick.

Then we added the "safety catch," which was:

My whole body is supple and flexible. I dance effortlessly and safely.

We did a single round of tapping for the goal, and a single round for the safety catch. He then performed three battements followed by three grande battement kicks. Here are the results:

Battement before EFT: 45.75 inches

Battement after EFT: 56.5 inches

Improvement: 10.75 inches

Grande Battement before EFT: 58.25 inches

Grande Battement after EFT: 61.25 inches

Improvement: 3 inches

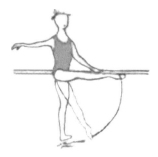

Battement Kick Height Limit

In the image above, the height I measured is the top of the right foot. This young athlete was quite amazed at the improvement since he's been working on improving these moves for several months and his initial kick height was the best he had been able to accomplish. Yet with EFT, he was immediately able to get large gains, and, with the safety catch, not risk a torn ligament in a very fast and strenuous move.

If I were working with an athlete intensively, I would look at the different muscle groups involved in the two kicks to determine why he got more improvement in the one kick than the other, then develop more targeted Setup Phrases for those particular muscles. The whole process with this young man took about 15 minutes, and I did not have time to develop the protocol for him further, since after watching him change, other family members wanted treatment with EFT!

❊ ❊ ❊

Many thanks to Lynn Francis of the U.K. for doing a detailed study while helping five golfers get over the "yips." This neuromuscular "jerking" problem affects not only golfers but baseball, basketball, and tennis players, dart throwers, and even dentists, musicians, and surgeons. For those who have them, the yips are a very serious problem.

EFT Eliminates Golfers' Yips

by Lynn Francis

The yips are a psycho-neuromuscular problem that often strikes golfers when they are putting but which can also affect them during other types of shots, whereby players experience freezing, jerking, or twitching immediately prior to impact. The movements they experience, which are involuntary (the affected person has no control over them), can add an average of 5.5 shots to a round.

Psychological responses include frustration, embarrassment, intense anxiety, and increased self-consciousness. Some golfers switch hands in an effort to prevent the yips, putting left-handed instead of right-handed, or vice versa. The longevity of the problem, which can last for years or decades, means that most golfers end up quitting. They cannot rationalize what is happening and they overanalyze what is going on.

The yips also affect other sports such as tennis and cricket darts (where it's commonly known as dartitis). Surgeons, dentists, and musicians can also suffer from the same type of involuntary movements.

So serious is the problem that the USA's Mayo Clinic conducted its own study to determine the cause, treatment, and cure.

Having worked with hundreds of cases using EFT for emotional issues, I decided to turn my attention to sports. I read all I could about the dreaded yips and found many theories as to the cause along with different treatments tried over the years. Although some claim to have cured the yips, none of the people I asked had any solid documented proof to back up their claim. This when I decided that I would try to cure the yips using EFT and, most importantly, get good documented proof of my work.

When I advertised in 2004 for golfers suffering with the yips to take part in a study, there was no shortage of volunteers. I chose a group of five based on their varying handicaps and ages, which ranged from professional golfer to double-figure handicap, the youngest being 28 and the oldest 59. I asked the players to write a lengthy report prior to treatment describing their symptoms and how the yips affected their game. After treatment they were asked to write a follow-up report.

I successfully cured all five of the cases using EFT by uncovering and eliminating emotional issues. Two years after the study concluded, I contacted all who took part and they all signed and dated a statement confirming that they are still yip-free to this present day.

What happened next was that Paul Chappell, editor of *Golfers Chronicle*, a magazine published in the U.K., reported the study. His article included the participating golfers' descriptions of their problems and their results.

Cliffe Grimshaw, age 59, had a 16 handicap. He had suffered from the yips for six years, especially on short putts and chips. "At first it showed itself as a jabbed stroke," he said, "but increasingly it developed with me freezing over the ball. It became difficult, even almost impossible, to draw back the putter. In trying to accommodate the problem I tried several different putters including the 'broomstick' type. I then started to putt with my left hand below my right. This still did not remove the problem, by which time it had also started to affect me while chipping the ball."

After learning and using EFT, he says, "The dread I used to feel when faced with these particular shots has gone. I no longer display the jabbing and freezing over the ball that I did prior to this treatment."

Next was Gerard Daly, age 42, with a 7 handicap. He suffered from the yips for two years on short putts. "My problem with the yips originally surfaced when it came to driving off the tee," he said. "I could not get the club back in the normal length of time. Eventually, the condition subsided after two or three months. Last year I started suffering the same, this time with my putting. As soon as I have a putt of 10 feet or less, I have an uncontrollable turn of my wrist. The shorter the putt, the more likely I am to push or pull it. The lengths I have gone to in order to eradicate this problem include using four different putters, shortening a putter, and changing my grip. But still the problem persists."

After using EFT, he reported, "Lynn has eliminated my yips problem completely. My game has improved to the extent that, rather than fear a six-foot or less putt, I now look forward with confidence in my ability to hole them on most if not all occasions."

Golfer Philip Leaver, age 41, had a 5 handicap. He suffered from the yips for five to six years while chipping and long-putting. "Nearly four years ago I started to suffer the yips while chipping around the greens," he said. "No matter how much I practiced, it showed no signs of abating. It arose only in pressure situations, for instance, if I needed to chip over a bunker to a tight pin location. My arm would stiffen and this caused me to thin the shot. This spring I also started to demonstrate the yips while putting."

After learning EFT, he said, "Since having the treatment I feel like I have been cured from an illness. My chipping has improved to a level where I now feel comfortable with any kind of pitch shot. Lynn has also worked on my putting problem which showed up on six- or seven-foot putts. My old stroke is back and I'm at ease with myself again."

Gareth Bradley, age 40, was a scratch handicapper from the Bramhall Golf Club. The yips had affected him for six years while chipping and long-putting. "The problem has been progressively getting worse from about 10 years ago," he said, "developing from the odd poor chip to much more. In the past two or three years the problem has crept into my longer putting. I am still OK with short putts. The frustration it is bringing is starting to become difficult to cope with and could possibly lead to me giving up the game.

"After just two sessions with Lynn, she appears to have completely eliminated the problem. I have played 17 competitive rounds since the sessions and have had no yips. The dread I used to feel before chipping has gone. Yes, I have hit some bad chips but these were down to poor technique and not a yip. My game is rejuvenated and I'm enjoying the game again."

The fifth participant was Jason Hartley, a 28-year-old professional golfer originally from South Africa and currently in Hertfordshire. He suffered from the yips for 12 years and it affected most of his shots. He said, "I first experienced the yips in 1992 at the age of 16. I was playing in a provincial tournament in South Africa. I remember walking up to a putt of about eight feet, feeling confident. I went through my normal routine but when I tried to make the putt, my hands seemed to jump just before I made contact with the ball.

"A little confused, I walked up to my remaining putt (above one foot in length) and did exactly the same thing again. Gradually it became worse. After struggling for a year I swapped from putting left-handed to putting right-handed, which I still do today. When I try and putt left-handed, I get a pins-

and-needles feeling all down my right arm. In the last two years the yip is developing in the rest of my game from a short chip to a drive. I find it hard to believe that the hands have time to twitch when the club is being swung at 125 miles an hour. I am terrified of actually hitting the ball. I need to sort this out as soon as possible as the game is becoming a chore and my confidence is at an all-time low. Just the thought of playing golf gives me that tingling feeling in my right side and I know my full swing is taking the same route as my putting did when it all started."

After learning EFT he wrote, "I still find it hard to believe that something that was so ingrained could be cured over the space of a few hours. Since seeing Lynn, my confidence is at an all-time high and I have started looking forward to playing again, and my scores are reflecting this. People who have never experienced the yips find the subject hard to comprehend, but for people who have and do, it is good to know that there is finally a definite cure."

A year later, the magazine published a follow-up article that described a second study that I conducted at the invitation of Mike Rotheram and Dr. Mark Bawden, researchers at Sheffield Hallam University.

One of the participants in their test was 50-year-old golfer Nigel Grice, who had a 5 handicap after learning to putt left-handed. He wished to switch back to right-handed putting.

When reporting into the laboratory for his baseline test, Nigel said, "I have suffered from the yips since the end of the 1999 season, when during a matchplay singles knockout semi-final competition, I missed about six very short putts due to what I can only describe as an electric shock in my left forearm. This caused the putter head to move involuntarily, leading to the putt being hopelessly missed." After that, Nigel was unable to putt and even broke down in tears at one point, due to the disintegration of his short game.

Nigel was required to take part in five data collections at the University following the EFT treatments I administered. All measurements were recorded when putting at a distance of two feet from the cup, where the yips tend to be at their most severe. Measures included a behavioral assessment (whether I could see the jerk) and self-report (Nigel's self-assessment). In addition, the researchers used the latest golf putting technology from SAM Motion Analysis, which measures the yips in golfers.

Of particular interest to Mike and Mark's study was the velocity of rotation as Nigel jerked the putter at impact. The results show that EFT was effective. All four measures improved dramatically from baseline scores. Behavioral assessment of the putting stroke added support to the findings.

Before the treatment, yipping occurred about 70 percent of the time. After the final treatment, there were no visual indicators of a yip occurring.

At the start of the study, Nigel reported the yip at maximum intensity when performing in the laboratory. However, after the final measurement, there now were no feelings of the yip at all. Mike asked Nigel to perform out on the golf course, and again there was no evidence of the yip occurring.

Nigel added, "The start of every golf season was always terrifying for me, as I never knew how much worse the yips had become, but now I look forward to the 2006 season with much excitement, fully confident that this terrible affliction has been finally exorcised by Lynn's exceptional skills and ability. I also believe that, as a bonus to curing the yips, I am now a different person. I see things and react differently to situations in everyday life. I feel better. I know that this is as a direct result of the therapy I underwent and would recommend it to anyone."

At the end of the study, Mike concluded, "Lynn's work is based on her skills as a practitioner in finding underlying emotional causes. The benefits of this treatment are not only relevant to amateur golfers. They are also relevant to tour players who experience the yips and people in other sports such as darts and cricket. Lynn has stumbled on something here that is potentially ground-breaking. This is undoubtedly the most effective treatment I have seen so far. It is now up to the scientific community to put these findings into appropriate research settings."

* * *

Before we leave the subject of statistics, here are some insights from Stacey Vornbrock, who uses EFT with elite and amateur athletes to release mental, emotional, physical, and mechanical blocks. She provides us with an illuminating description of the true progress that athletes most prefer, raising some interesting points about EFT benefits that may not be reflected in a player's statistics.

What Is an Athlete Really Looking to Improve?

by Stacey Vornbrock

I feel compelled to address some beliefs and hypotheses I've seen put forth about statistical results of using EFT for improved sports performance. I've been breaking new ground by taking EFT to professional athletes since 2003 and feel the need to share what I am discovering, which is very different from some of the common hypotheses. I think heading down the path of relating EFT to statistical performance results unnecessarily sets up EFT practitioners to feel as though they have failed.

I know because for the first two years of my EFT practice, I felt I had failed my athletes because the statistical results that I thought I should see weren't there. However, all my athletes were reporting great results and were very happy with what EFT had done for them. I was the one who wasn't happy because I thought something else should be happening. Let me clarify this.

There isn't one professional or amateur athlete who has come to me wanting a statistical result of any kind. Not one athlete has come to increase his batting average, take a stroke or two off his game, kick further, or throw further. They have all come to have their mental and emotional blocks removed because they know that once those blocks are gone, they will absolutely perform at their highest level, whatever it is.

They come to improve their focus and mental discipline and to address their anxiety, loss of confidence, fear of re-injury, recovery from injuries, loss of range of motion, past performance trauma, mechanical challenges, fear and doubt, stress, relief from pain, and lack of consistency.

Here's what one of my Olympic athletes said about EFT: "Tapping doesn't make me a better athlete. Tapping frees me to be a better athlete. There is a correlation between tapping and having a clear state of mind. Tapping frees me up to throw further and it frees me up to focus. Tapping has given me the possibility of reaching my full potential."

EFT didn't cause my college football kicker to kick his 46- and 47-yard field goals. He could kick 60-yard field goals in practice. EFT removed the blocks so he could succeed in a game under pressure. This is true for all my guys. EFT simply removed the blocks that prevented them from performing at their highest level, whatever that is. The highest level isn't the same for every athlete. Not every athlete has the talent to win. Not every athlete has the talent to have a high batting average or set records in his or her sport.

There are two major areas that factor into an athlete's statistical success. The first has to do with all the issues mentioned above, such as injuries, anxiety, loss of confidence, etc. This is the area that EFT can have a big impact on. I have had great success in removing all of those blocks.

The second area involves factors that EFT and I can't control and which affect success. These include the athletes' level of talent; their commitment to practice; whether they continue to tap as needed; their nutrition (many athletes have very poor nutritional habits); competition conditions; weather; and the talent they play against. This last area plays a much larger factor in statistical results.

Whenever we attach EFT to an athlete's statistical results, we severely short-change the power of EFT because when the stats go down (and they will fluctuate) it looks as though EFT isn't working anymore or that EFT failed. What's sad is that by continuing to focus on statistical results, we miss the really big news about what EFT can do for athletes, and that is remove all the blocks that keep them from performing at their highest level.

Here's what I can report statistically about the athletes that I've worked with:

- 100 percent eliminated or significantly reduced their anxiety so it is no longer an issue when they play their sport.

- 100 percent reported improved confidence.

- 100 percent no longer re-injured body parts that were injured.

- 100 percent completed the healing of old injuries.

- 100 percent sped up the healing of current injuries.

- 100 percent increased their range of motion by at least 20 percent and often much more (a 10-percent increase is considered outstanding).

- 100 percent cleared up their past performance traumas.

- 100 percent made mechanical changes within minutes during a session.

- 100 percent released doubt and fear about their performance issues.

- 100 percent reported relief from pain, in most cases the complete elimination of pain.

- 100 percent improved their consistency in their performance.

- 100 percent significantly improved their ability to focus while performing.

- 100 percent improved their mental discipline.

This is *huge* news. There isn't any other tool or technique out there that I'm aware of that can produce results like this. There isn't anyone talking to athletes about clearing all these blocks for them because they can't. Only EFT can do that. The big news isn't about EFT producing statistical results. The big news is that EFT removes blocks that nothing else does.

In the world of golf, there are numerous clubs and pieces of equipment that promise to take strokes off your game. But no one is saying to these golfers, "I can eliminate or significantly reduce your anxiety on the golf course. I can increase your range of motion so you are more fluid in your swing. I can clear out all those bad shots you've made in the past. I can help you make mechanical changes in your swing in minutes as opposed to years."

In the world of baseball, there are coaches who help players with their batting averages or Earned Run Averages (ERAs). But no one is saying to these ball players, "I can totally eliminate your fear of re-injury. I can help you manage your adrenaline on the field. I can help your body make a quick physical recovery after the game so you feel ready to play the next night. I can help you increase your focus at bat so you can clearly see the ball come out of the pitcher's hand."

This is the really big news and these are the issues that athletes want help with. They aren't identifying statistical results as the problem because they all know that once their blocks are removed, the statistics will take care of themselves. Let's start focusing on the real benefits of EFT and sports performance, which are that EFT can remove mental, emotional, physical, and mechanical blocks so that athletes can perform at their highest level possible, whatever that is, based on their talent, commitment to practice, nutritional practices, competition conditions, and the skill of their opponents.

❁ ❁ ❁

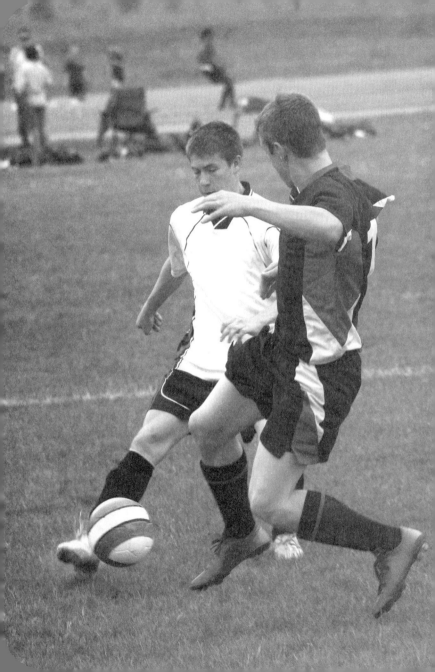

4

EFT and
Championships

Whether we're talking about team sports or individual competitions, the right mental/emotional preparation makes all the difference. Here are some great examples from people who used EFT to improve their chances at the championship level.

Stephanie Drieze, a professional Social Worker and "Little League Baseball Mom," successfully applied EFT to the various baseball issues confronting her son and other team members. As you will see, the field is a great place for athletes to address all aspects of life. This goes for all athletes, from Little League to the Olympics.

Stephanie refers at one point to the 9 Gamut Procedure. This technique is part of EFT's original Basic Recipe but not the shortcut version described in Chapter One. You'll find it described in Appendix A.

EFT "Field of Dreams"—Little League Baseball

by Stephanie Drieze

This is an account of how I used EFT with the children on a struggling Little League baseball team. The players were 10, 11, and 12 years old. Early in the season, it became apparent to my husband, the team's manager, that the concentration of talent was limited to only a few players, which made winning or even competing in games quite difficult! After five consecutive losses, he asked me to intervene and work with a few of the players, with consent from the players and their parents, to see if it would help the team's overall situation.

I started with my older son, "B." Although "B" is a very strong baseball player, he hadn't played well consistently in the early games. He tapped on:

Even though I feel this pressure, I deeply and completely accept myself.

Even though I step out of the batter's box...

In the first game he played after tapping on these issues, he hit his first big home run out of the park!

I then worked with "H," a pitcher who was struggling with anger at his teammates for their fielding errors. He subsequently pitched a strong, confident game, with lots of strike-outs. From then on, "H" insisted on tapping before all games. After one tapping session, he pitched against the best-hitting team in the league and threw a *No Hitter!*

[*My comment:* In case you are not "baseball savvy," a No Hitter is a superb pitching accomplishment at any age. It means no other opposing player got to first base by getting a base hit.]

I was asked by several of the players' parents to work with their children on whatever their baseball issues were. The players were able to articulate their concerns quite well once they started tapping. One player tapped on his habit of stepping out of the batter's box during a pitch, but during the course of the session he said, *"No, wait, it's actually that I'm afraid of getting hit by the pitch."* So, we tapped on his fear of being hit by the ball. All of the players who tapped were able to rate their emotional block or problem before and after each round of tapping.

One of the players came to learn the tapping technique but through talking with his mother, I learned that he actually had been diagnosed with an anxiety disorder and that baseball was simply one of his many crippling worries.

The mother gave me permission to work with "L" on all his fears, which included being afraid of failing a test; throwing up; having trouble breathing; and not being able to sleep through the night. Interestingly, this boy did not experience much relief from several rounds of the shortcut Basic Recipe, so I suggested the 9 Gamut Procedure. One round with the 9 Gamut Procedure and his fear went to zero. His mother, who was watching asked him if it was really a zero, although we both could visually see a huge shift in his body language. He replied, *"Mum, it's actually zero. Zero!"* At that point the mother and I were both crying!

My husband said that "L" was a different, more confident, and happier player at practice that night, joking and "in the game". I saw "L" one more time to reinforce his positive gains and he was in excellent shape. The mother said she and he tap at night together and he hadn't had any problems sleeping, had gone to school every day, and felt like "his old, normal self."

A related vignette regarding another player, "D," occurred well after baseball season ended. He was playing at our home when an intense thunderstorm passed through quickly with lots of lightning, wind, and even dime-sized hail. I remembered that "D" had always been afraid of thunderstorms and usually hid in the basement or a bathroom whenever and wherever one struck. I looked for "D" and when I found him, he was coming up the basement stairs with a big smile on his face. I asked him if he was OK and he said *"I am now, Mrs. Drieze; I just did the tapping."* He was using EFT on his own, and he told me that he uses it whenever a situation "needs the tapping!"

In the end, we didn't win the championship, but the team played very well the rest of the season. The players improved significantly and seemed to enjoy the Little League experience more. All the players who engaged in the tapping technique with me experienced real, physical relief of symptoms and played baseball more confidently, with significantly reduced anxiety, enhanced performance, and greater desire.

✽ ✽ ✽

Gina Parris gives us a good example of how EFT can improve athletic performance when she focuses on her son's batting form in baseball. Her report includes an excellent example of how to use affirmations and the tail-enders they produce to create effective EFT Setups, a concept described in Chapter Two.

EFT and a Baseball State Championship

by Gina Parris

My son Jordan was a weak batter in his beloved game of baseball. Very often he made the final out of the inning, and he hated that. He had a fear of hitting the ball into the dirt or popping it up and getting thrown out at first. His body simply cooperated to fulfill his anxieties.

During our first EFT session, he realized that in his mind, he had never been a power hitter. He believed that no one thought he could hit, including himself. His at-bats simply fulfilled his beliefs, even though he tried to stay positive.

Jordan also made the connection that the college girls he had just watched on TV could hit a ball out of the park because of their form, not their size, so he could choose to hit with perfect form and hit as well as anybody. This was important, because Jordan is a bit more slender than some of his teammates. Jordan's new thoughts alone though, were not enough. After all, he had made these kinds of observations before.

Before, when trying to be positive, he would tell himself, "I'm going to get a hit, I'm going to get a hit…" but his mind would argue through images of past pop-ups and weak grounders, and the resulting state was one of conflict and doubt.

So we tapped on his self-image of being a weak batter. We tapped on what it takes to be a power hitter. We tapped on how to choose perfect form. Just an hour after our session, he went back to the park where he and his coach worked on his batting form before the game.

In that game, for the first time ever, "skinny Jordan" confidently stepped up to the plate and sent the outfielders scrambling as he hit the ball to the fence! Then he got another hit and another, before finally drawing a walk. His at-bats brought in five runs and the team enjoyed a handy victory. More importantly, his hitting remained strong after that, and he went on to use the technique to improve his defense as well. His whole season was marked by amazing improvement.

It is interesting to note that it often takes hundreds of swings to correct one's batting form, but we have seen many examples where an athlete was able to correct his form in one day with EFT tapping. This also applies to golf swings, pitching form, free throws, and other athletics.

The important thing to see here is that Jordan needed time to focus on his distressing thoughts — weak grounders and pop-ups — and clear out their ability to mess up his form. He also needed to be prepared to execute the perfect form that his coach showed him.

Today, most of the time, if Jordan is at bat and has an image of hitting a weak grounder, his automatic response is to hit with perfect form. In fact, most everything about the at-bat triggers a response of "perfect form." Do you see how this would turn any batter into a confident and reliable hitter?

Jordan's teammates were so impressed with his performance that he finally shared his "secret" with all of them. He knew that if they all tapped, they could come out of obscurity and win the State Championship. Indeed, that is exactly what happened. The little team that played in the state tournament only because they were hosting it started tapping with me before each game, and they totally dominated the event. In the newspaper coverage that followed, the headline read, "State Champs Had Secret Weapon." To you and me, it's no secret.

※ ※ ※

Laura Campbell reports on an apparent EFT-inspired athletic improvement of her daughter's soccer team. As she demonstrates, the emotional/mental component is often the difference between winning and losing. Laura mentions the 9 Gamut Procedure, which is described in Appendix A.

Soccer Performance—EFT or Coincidence?

by Laura Campbell

My 12-year-old daughter plays soccer on a fairly new team. They played in a tournament this weekend. My daughter hurt her leg in the first game Saturday, so I was trying to get her to tap on it. She was embarrassed in front of her friends, but one of them asked me to show her how to do it. All the girls were sitting on the ground in front of me and as I demonstrated for one, they all began to tap.

Their next game was against a team that usually beats them by eight or nine points, and in soccer, that's a slaughter. Some of them were intimidated prior to tapping. At half-time, they were ahead 1-0. During the second half, my daughter yelled at me, "Mom, we tapped and we're winning." She later told me they even tapped at half-time. All the parents were raving about how great the girls were playing. They lost the game 2-1, but they never gave up and played with "heart."

They tapped before their first game on Sunday and won. They had 15 minutes before they had to play an undefeated team in First Place in the tournament. The coach even asked me to do that "meditation thing you did" before the game. I led them in tapping for their tension and sore muscles and then for their best performance. I included the 9 Gamut Procedure to help them focus. They played another excellent game, never gave up, and lost by only two scores.

Did EFT make a difference? I think so. They all played better than I've seen them play, with fewer mistakes and better coordination. They got their foot on the ball, ran hard, and had fun! Granted, this is not scientific evidence, but it's interesting!

❊ ❊ ❊

Brent Thomson, PhD, has used EFT on many occasions to dramatically improve sports performance. He gives us details here as he describes his impressive work with a high school girls basketball team. Please note how he isolates the issues involved. Getting to individual issues like this often spells the difference between good results and spectacular results. All athletes have their individualized beliefs, idiosyncracies, and other barriers to achieving their full potential.

Also note that the basketball team, among other achievements, improved their free throw percentage by a mammoth 87 percent.

EFT for a High School Basketball Team
by Brent Thomson, Ph.D.

I recently worked with the entire Red Wing High School Girls Basketball team in Red Wing, Minnesota, using EFT to improve team performance. I met with the team for a two-hour session. At that time their record was five games below the 500 mark.

Historically, the girls' team has struggled, usually winning anywhere from three to five games in a year. We talked with the team members and the coaching staff and came up with the following "hit" list of problems that needed to be chopped down: *Poor free throw shooting. Poor jump shooting. Poor use of the clock. Losing focus and concentration. Poor passing. Fear of making mistakes. Consistently playing below ability level. Easily intimidated by the other team. Easily affected by crowd noise.*

We put each of these in the familiar *"Even though"* format and proceeded to tap on each one. We did three or four rounds on each issue and then talked about other issues that surfaced. What I found by doing this is that specific issues started to surface for each of the players and we were then able to isolate those and tap them down on an individual basis.

I also found that the team really enjoyed doing the tapping "as a team." A number of the players and coaches noted a general sense of purpose, and a positive sense of team unity was a side effect of the group tapping.

We kept track of the statistics in terms of free throw percentage as a team before tapping and again after tapping. Also, we kept records of shooting percentages, both before and after tapping.

Overall, the team has improved 87 percent in free throw shooting percentage since tapping. Before tapping, they were making a dismal 40 out of 100 as a team. Since applying EFT the team has played eight games and in those eight games they skyrocketed to a team average of 75 out of 100.

Overall shooting averages for the eight games previous to tapping was 37 out of 100. Shooting percentage in the last eight games since the EFT session is now 54 out of 100. That's a 46-percent improvement.

Their record in the last eight games is six wins and only two losses. One of the losses was by only three points to a team ranked in the top five in the State of Minnesota. Earlier that year, before EFT, they were blown out by over 30 points.

Both the coaching staff and the players attribute the improvement to the addition of EFT to their training procedures. I am convinced EFT has a significant place in training individual athletes and teams so that they can maximize their physical abilities and play with greater stamina, speed, strength, and coordination.

❖ ❖ ❖

High school competitions are a serious business, and with their high stakes come the same emotional blocks that can impair professional athletes. In this next report, Brent Thomson helps the captain of a high school gymnastics team recover mentally and emotionally from an ankle injury.

EFT for a High School Gymnast
by Brent Thomson, Ph.D.

I recently had the opportunity to work with, Katie Auge, the captain of her high school gymnastics team in Red Wing, Minnesota, which is where I live. She has been struggling this year with a nagging ankle injury and has been receiving physical therapy on an ongoing basis. The injury has significantly affected her scoring as well as her overall confidence throughout the year.

Katie is a senior and her wish is to make the state gymnastics meet in the All Around Competition. Her dad called to ask if I would work with her. I had done so her last year, during her junior year, on three occasions, and she really enjoyed EFT. She had never made the state tournament previously.

I met with her for one session the day of the regional meet that would decide whether or not she would go on to the state competition. The meet was held at her high school, so many friends and relatives would be watching.

We tapped on the following:

Even though I'm afraid of falling and hurting myself on the vault, I deeply and completely accept myself.

Even though I'm worried about my ankle holding up in the competition today...

Even though I have all this anxiety about performing well in front of friends and family...

Even though I have this fear of failure...

Even though I have fears about sticking the landing on the vault...

The session was 90 minutes long. We were able to get her anxiety about all of the aforementioned targets down to zero on the 0-to-10 intensity scale. Katie concluded her session with:

I choose to see myself performing in a graceful, relaxed, confident, and powerful manner in all my events today.

Katie didn't completely believe this statement at first, but after tapping on it for four rounds, she rated her belief of it at a 9.

Gary is always looking for statistics to indicate proof that EFT works, and I have some. I received a call on Saturday morning from a very excited Katie and her father saying she "nailed" the vault and qualified for her first state competition in the All Around Competition category.

Katie says that there is no doubt that the EFT was the strategy that put her over the top. In addition, she said that her ankle did not bother her at all during the meet, and that her confidence was consistently high. She attributes this to the EFT work we did on the day of the regional meet. Think what we could have accomplished if we had a little more training time!

* * *

This next article, which was submitted by John Freedom on behalf of his client, Tammy Bredy, is a glowing example of the mental game that directs physical outcomes. Note how many issues are successfully resolved and how, when simple tapping doesn't immediately clear a problem, John and Tammy search for specific events from the past that are somehow linked to present emotions. Once the emotional charge from an old (and often buried) memory has been neutralized, it no longer contributes to the problem.

Woman Archer Wins Gold Medal with EFT

by John Freedom

Tammy Bredy is a mom, massage therapist, and archer who lives in Cedar Crest, New Mexico. She learned EFT at an EFT training workshop and two weeks later participated in her first archery shoot. Here is her account of how she used EFT to win her first two competitions and come in second place at the third, competing against some of the best archers in the country, including native Navajos who'd been shooting arrows since childhood, all under extreme conditions. This long report clearly illustrates the ways in which EFT can be applied before, during, and after a sports event.

Here is Tammy's report:

My first shoot was in Red River, New Mexico. I was very nervous about going to a competition at the level of "State Qualifying." I decided to go for the experience and the practice. The course was harder than I had ever shot. There were a lot of long-range shots. Many of them were up steep hills, down steep hills, and over gullies and streams. In lots of shots the arrow had to thread between branches.

I started feeling like I didn't belong there. I wasn't good enough to be there. I was a "new shooter." I started tapping, saying:

Even though I'm a new shooter, I deeply and completely accept myself.

Even though I don't think I can compete at this level…

Even though I'm not "good enough"…

Even though I may not judge the distance correctly…

Even though I don't always hold my bow just right…

I tapped as we walked to the next target. I made sure I was walking behind the group. While tapping, my head became very clear, and I calmed down. Some long shots were next. My arrows flew just right and hit the scoring rings. I felt good about the shots but still had doubts about keeping up the good shots. I tapped on my doubt:

Even though I doubt my ability, I deeply and completely accept myself.

Even though I still don't think I am "good enough"…

Even though I am shooting with these "experts"…

Even though I don't think I can keep up…

I kept shooting well. I felt happy and gained some confidence. I kept doing EFT the rest of the day.

Even though I don't always hold my bow in exactly the right place…

Even though I don't always line my peep up just right…

Even though I sometimes shoot too quickly…

Even though I drop my bow too quickly…

Even though my arm gets tired…

When the scores were posted, I was 24 points ahead of the second-place person! The next day I came to the shoot thinking the day before was just "lucky." I still wasn't really that good an archer. I tapped on the doubt again:

Even though I doubt my shooting skills, I deeply and completely accept myself.

Even though I am not really "that good"….

Even though I think yesterday was "just a fluke"….

I shot the first eight targets very well and received high scores. At this point I started tapping for the opposite of my problem statements.

I am a good archer.

My arrows will fly perfectly.

I am not dropping my bow early.

I am lining the peep up perfectly.

I am releasing my string just right.

My arm is not shaking. I am perfectly still.

I will not move till I hear the arrow hit.

I am choosing the bull's eye every shot.

I kept shooting well and started to really enjoy being there. I won the shoot (this was my first competition!) and was very pleased.

My second shoot was a bigger challenge because it was held on an Indian reservation in New Mexico on a very hot day. I do not do well in the heat. I started tapping right away:

Even though I'm not sure why I came to this shoot, I deeply and completely accept myself.

Even though I don't do well in the heat…

Even though I did well at the first shoot…

Even though I will make friends with the heat for these two days…

Even though the heat will not affect my shooting…

Even though my body will keep the heat away from my body's boundaries…

Even though I am shooting with Navajos whose traditions include archery…

The targets were in crevices of rocks. The ground was harder. I knew my body would be drained after walking on this terrain in the New Mexico heat in July.

Even though this day will be taxing on my body….

…I will hydrate and keep focused.

…I will enjoy my walk.

…I will enjoy walking with my fellow archers and being with them.

…I will BE ALL HERE and keep my mind on the shoot only.

...I will do all the right steps I know to do to make good shots.

My legs started feeling "heavy" and tired. I tapped on:

I feel light.

I know I am strong.

I know I have practiced.

I know I can hit the bull's eye.

I know my arrows can fly well, and will.

I started feeling better and happier and I enjoyed the shoot. I won this shoot as well and went away this time thinking I was going to keep being a good archer.

My third shoot was near Shiprock in the Four Corners area of northern Arizona. It was very hot, over 100° Fahrenheit (38° Celsius) and also involved walking a canyon and up and down rocks. I was competing against native Navajos, who learn to shoot while still children and are some of the best archers in the country. I began the shoot, making good shots. Then my stomach started hurting again. I had had a stomachache and flu feelings the day before but thought it was over. It turned out to be a flu that lasted a day after the shoot. My head was also hurting. I started shooting poorly and keep shooting poorly this first round. I started tapping:

Even though I have started this shoot off poorly, I deeply and completely accept myself.

Even though I am shooting with some of the best archers in the country...

Even though I am feeling sick...

Even though I am having trouble focusing...

Even though it is getting very hot...

Even though my first round wasn't a good score, and I was SICK...

...I can learn from these Navajo archers.

...I can still have fun.

...this can still be a good day.

...my stomach will feel better and my head will stop hurting.

...this bug I am fighting will not pull me down.

...my body can endure this shoot and I can rise above this.

...I will not drop my bow.

...I will line up my peep.

...I will judge the distance properly.

...I will not rush my shots.

My second round score was much better. My body was feeling weak, but no longer feeling sick. I tapped on:

My arrows will fly with ease like eagles.

I can make it through this shoot.

I can finish and do well.

I can be all present for this shoot.

I imagined light clearing my body again. I was doing well this last round.

I will feel good the rest of this shoot.

I will learn from my fellow archers, and enjoy the rest of this shoot.

My stamina will hold out.

I will keep my focus.

I will not get anxious.

I will not drop my bow.

The heat will not affect my shooting.

I will stay focused till the last target is shot.

This round was great! I scored very high. I wasn't going to turn my score card in, but I did. I placed second and was surprised that my score was as good as it was, given what the conditions were and how sick I had felt at first. EFT made all the difference,

John Freedom continues:

I did some more work with Tammy recently. I asked her what was a problem for her, and she said that she felt impatient and was rushing her shots. We tapped on "feeling impatient," which got lighter, but there was still something there. "Why are you rushing your shots?" I asked. She replied, "I feel like I shouldn't keep people waiting." I asked her, "When you were a little girl, who used to rush you, and who told you that you were keeping people waiting?" She thought a moment, and then looked down and grimaced. "My stepdad. He was always impatient with me." We did another round of tapping after using these Setups:

> *Even though my stepdad was always rushing me, I deeply and completely accept myself.*
>
> *Even though my stepdad was always on my case…*
>
> *Even though my stepdad blamed me and shamed me…*
>
> *Even though I felt like I shouldn't keep people waiting…*
>
> *I know that was about HIM and not about me.*
>
> *I know that that was then, and this is NOW.*
>
> *I know that I'm a strong, powerful adult now.*
>
> *I can TAKE AS MUCH TIME AS I NEED.*
>
> *And I can relax, pick my shots, and enjoy myself, whether I win or lose.*
>
> *And I'm choosing to relax, take my time, and do the best I can.*

We then alternated tapping on feeling impatient, feeling rushed, not keeping people waiting, and feeling calm, having plenty of time, taking her time, etc.

After several rounds of tapping, I asked her if there was anything else. She thought a moment and said, "I'm feeling self-conscious because I'll be competing with a hunting bow. Most of the archers will be using performance bows, which are more expensive, easier to draw, and more accurate. My hunting bow is heavier and more difficult to draw."

"What do you feel when you think of competing against these other archers with a hunting bow?"

She hung her head and said, "I feel like I'm at a disadvantage, and like I'm less than."

Tammy had grown up poor in rural Wyoming and often wore hand-me-downs. Even though her family could have bought good clothes for her, her stepfather refused to spend any money on her. She got a job when she was 12 years old so that she could buy decent clothes for herself. Having an "inferior" bow compared to the other archers was plugging her into the shame and deprivation of her childhood. I decided to help her use this to her advantage.

Even though I'm competing with a hunting bow, when the other archers will have performance bows, I deeply and completely accept myself.

Even though I'm feeling defective and less-than, like I did when I was a child…

Even though I feel handicapped and like I'm at a disadvantage…

I know that I've had to work harder than others all my life, and that has made me strong.

I know that I'm very competitive, and I do my best when competing.

I know that I've been "at a disadvantage" my whole life, and this has only made me stronger.

I'm putting my best foot forward, doing the best I can, and que sera, sera.

*I can tap on myself, release these old inade-
quate feelings, and discover how adequate and capable I
really am.*

*I'm choosing to take my time, work with what I
have, and do the best I can.*

Tammy says, "In the morning I was red hot, I
could not miss, but then I got really tired later that
day. I was starting to wear out and was not shooting
as well. I tried to figure out what was going on. I was
trying different things. This other gal had gained a
few points on me. I thought the game was over, but
we had one more target, a javelina target. My husband had bought me a javelina, the same 3D target. I
told myself, 'I know I can make this shot.' I took my
time, waited until I was totally ready, and hit the dead
center of the bull's eye. It was a photo finish."

Tammy Bredy took first place in the New Mexico
games in June. The next month she competed in the
Western States Games in Colorado Springs, an event
that brings hundreds of athletes in virtually all sports
together. Competing against archers from all over the
country, she won the gold medal in the 3D competition and silver in the target competition. This was only
her second year of competing and the first time she
had competed in the Western States Competition.

❖ ❖ ❖

Peter Guare, an Albany, New York, high school track
coach, helped one of his athletes impressively improve his
performance. Notice the many uses of EFT in his report.

EFT Helps Track Star Win Three Gold Medals

by Peter Guare

I'm a Personal Performance Coach making the transition from Head Track Coach at a high school. Although I no longer get paid, I still help out with the program. I was working with Mike Tamul and some other hurdlers and showed them how to improve their flexibility, which is a must for hurdlers.

We used the Setup Phrase:

Even though I have this tension in my back and legs, I deeply and completely accept myself.

Tapping the sequence of EFT points, we used the Reminder Phrases *"tension in the muscles," "tension in the joints," "tension in the fascia," "tension in the ligaments,"* etc. When everyone improved markedly, they became converts. But Mike really heeded my advice and used it for everything, from making his trail leg faster in the hurdles to reducing pain and fatigue in the 1500 meters, an event in the pentathlon. I'll let him tell the rest of the story.

"My senior year is where I really began to excel," says Mike. "Mr. Guare taught me a tapping technique that could be used anywhere at any time and which could really help not only in Track but in many areas of life.

"This technique brought a new level of focus to me and increased my flexibility quickly. After only a week or two, I found myself at an invitational in ugly weather. Before all of my races, I tapped and

I focused on winning. That meet I accomplished something I had never done before: I won three gold medals.

"I became a Sectional Champion in the 110 Meter High Hurdles with the help of Mr. Guare. The whole season we had actually been training hurdles for the pentathlon that I hoped to compete in at the New York State Championship meet. My time improved enough to add points to my pentathlon score and break the school record for that event.

"My score allowed me to compete at the State meet, where I placed fifth in the pentathlon. Mr. Guare's techniques helped me gain a winning mentality. I was eventually able to tap mentally during my 1500-meter race in the pentathlon and I was more relaxed and focused than ever, beating my record from the previous year by 17 seconds."

❉ ❉ ❉

Thanks to Jan Scholtes of the Netherlands for describing the intricate details behind EFT's use for a well known world-class athlete. You will find that celebrities and star athletes have issues just like everyone else and it is the collapsing of these issues that frees them to perform at top levels.

EFT and a World Pole-vaulting Championship

by Jan Scholtes

I have known pole-vaulter Rens Blom for many years and we see each other several times a year. He learned his basic techniques about how to get the proper relaxation at the right moments and we knew the importance of his thoughts during his preparations and during the games. But after I learned about EFT, we had more tools for handling his obstructive thoughts.

I had him keep a diary of his activities and thoughts during his preparations on the day of the match. In this diary I read a lot of doubts about his condition, doubts about how to behave as a sportsman, doubts about which pole to use, and doubts about things which could go wrong. These were not the thoughts of a champion who believed in himself. These were the thoughts of a boy who was doubting all day and was very easy influenced by things that happened around him. His thoughts were always sticking on the scenario of failure.

I taught him the EFT tapping techniques, which he thought was pretty strange. We tapped on his doubts and things that always went wrong during important tournaments, like:

Even though I feel very doubtful and afraid of making the wrong decisions, I deeply and completely accept myself.

I asked him what would be his biggest problem about making the wrong decisions. After a moment of reflection he looked at me and said. "I get anxious about the tone of the journalists and the critics when they comment on my way of jumping."

When I asked him if this reminded him of criticism he experienced before in his life, he remembered a trainer in his youth who very often had an authoritarian air which brought up feelings of resistance in him. I asked, "What's bothering you so much about people who act like an authority?" Rens answered, "It's often the tone of their voice that makes me feel guilty, as if I deserve punishment and I hate that." It also reminded him of his father, a disciplined man who had been a great sportsman, too, and whose tone of voice had a lot of temper. "He's a good-hearted man," Rens said, "and he supports me everywhere I go, but when I was younger he could have been more helpful."

After having said that we tapped on issues like;

Even though the tone of my father's voice is still in the back of my head, I deeply and completely accept myself.

Even though he always wanted me to do the things his way...

Even though I hate dominant men...

Even though I feel resistance against compelling ways of arguing...

Even though I have this problem with authority...

He felt relieved after bringing those feelings to his consciousness and tapping on them.

During an important competition, he failed his third effort at a certain height and showed a lot of frustration. "I gave 100 percent and I did my utmost," he tried to convince me. Because I was there and sensed something else, I asked him to very slowly review his thoughts during the time between his second jump and the start of his third effort. After about 20 seconds he glanced at me and said, "Shit. When I was sitting on the bank, I was preparing my excuses for the press." His game was already over.

From that he learned how important it is to consistently scan his negative thoughts, to be mentally aware, and to stay focused on the positive goal.

There was also the issue of breaking out of his comfort zone. He hadn't jumped a new personal record for two years and got frustrated about that. When I asked him if he had ever had a mental picture of seeing himself jumping to a new personal record, he remembered that he had tried but that those movies always ended in failure.

I had him visualize a movie in which he would jump to his new personal record (about 5 centimeters more, to keep it realistic for him). That wasn't easy for him because he kept seeing himself doing wrong jumps. I asked him if he could remember his best jump ever and how that felt. Of course he could; sportsman have those memories, same as they have strong memories about their failures. I asked him to use that positive state of mind in his new movie and let him try again. He had more luck this time and I asked him to train this way mentally while being aware that it was on personal-record level and to use an EFT statement like:

Even though I feel perfect jumping over 5.80, I deeply and completely accept myself.

Rens always preferred nice weather during the games. That's when he made his best jumps. In cold weather he always felt miserable, got cramps, and started complaining.

During the World Championships in Helsinki, Finland, this year, the weather was stormy, cold, and it rained cats and dogs. A nice scenario for Rens to prove that everything always goes wrong during important tournaments. But after the classifications, during which it stormed enormously, we had contact by email and I read the email of an athlete who had learned how to handle these conditions. I didn't read anything about doubts. I read about his chances and determination to do his outmost.

He was self-supporting now and used statements like:

Even though I hate bad weather, I deeply and completely accept myself.

Even though I hate these conditions and get distracted, I choose to accept them and handle them professionally.

During the finals he heard his fellow competitors yell and curse about the bad weather conditions and one after another they left the competition. That made him stronger in his determination to accept everything. He thought, *"OK, guys, spoil your energy on the weather. I stay by myself, I accept this weather, I am a professional, and I want to do my job."*

After Rens became World Champion, Serge Bubka, a Russian multi-champion vault jumper whom Rens idolized, gave him the biggest compliment he could get. He said he admired Rens for his courage and determination and that his strong character in those terrible weather conditions had made him a world champion.

And I was at home in front of the TV and saw it all happen. Who could have imagined years ago that this doubtful young man who possessed lots of videos of Serge Bubka would receive such a compliment from his hero? For me it was again proof that a lot is possible when the mind is free.

After the world games I was asked to help more athletes with their preparations for the next Olympic games. I met them last week and listened to their fears and failures and explained the importance of mental hygiene. In a group session we worked on several issues with individual athletes and the results where instant. One of them had an enormous experience of failure during the Olympic Games in Athens, which still troubled him during every match. After one session he felt relief from that. The expression on his face told the whole story. All of them felt strong relief from the problems they worked on and announced that they definitely wanted to continue. In individual talks with them I learned there is still a lot to do, but what an exciting challenge that is for me and for EFT.

❊ ❊ ❊

Here is an ideal case for those who are timid about trying EFT, especially on themselves. Lonnie Graf had these self-doubts regarding her use of EFT on a form of dancing stage fright. It was either that or experience panic during the performance.

Dancing with EFT

by Lonnie Graf

At 62, I have been taking ballroom lessons for the last year. I had never taken lessons or learned steps other than sixth-grade ballroom so finally took the leap and I'm so grateful that I did. This past Friday at an Arthur Awards Show, I was to perform my first routine, a combination Rumba/Argentine Tango. I knew the routine really well, but during my lesson Thursday afternoon, I felt my smile freeze, which was an indication to me that I was thinking about the spectators being there.

Then that night I kept waking up thinking about the performance. By Friday morning I was having a panic attack with the energy surging through my body. All I could think was there is no way I will be able to make it through my performance.

I had heard about EFT a year ago and had ordered the manual and many of the videos and thought it was awesome and shared it with others. And yet I only used it on myself once briefly. For some reason I didn't feel comfortable with my ability to use it even though it served me well in that brief period.

Well, Friday morning I received one of Gary's EFT newsletter emails and decided to check it out – and sure enough, there was a reference to how it had helped a woman who was afraid to dance.

Even though I know how to do EFT, I still didn't trust myself. I emailed a couple of people with a "help" request about doing a phone session for my performance that night. As I realized I might not hear back from anyone, I finally pulled myself together to do it for myself just in case. I did three rounds each set and I did three sets each hour for three hours and began to feel much calmer. Then I found I was beginning to look forward to the experience. I did one more set two hours before I left for good measure.

It was amazing how I was able to calm myself down to the point that I had no more anxiety. I felt really good during the evening and just before my performance I had that excited feeling with the edge to it which is so natural—but no racing heart, no utter fear. I had a great performance and felt really good about myself. My goal while doing EFT was to feel totally relaxed during my performance, to enjoy the experience, and to possibly even expand myself. It all happened! The judge seemed really impressed. The next day I had a critique with the judge where he rates your performance and he gave me a 95—my highest score—and he was unaware this was my first time to perform a routine. As an added bonus at the show, there were drawings for door prizes and I won the top prize of five dance lessons. I was flying high!

❊ ❊ ❊

EFT improves the performance of just about every athlete who takes it seriously. This includes Mark Ellis, who used EFT to bowl his first 300 game in over 30 years as a bowler. Notice how, during the game, Mark tapped mostly on his Karate Chop point, at times tapping the side of his hand against the ball return.

EFT and My Perfect Game

by Mark Ellis

I discovered EFT just over a year ago and I have been having great personal success with it for various pain issues and emotional well-being. I have always been intrigued by the stories of personal improvement for athletes but have not had the opportunity to try it for sports until recently.

I have been a league bowler for over 30 years and have steadily improved to the point where I have carried a 190–200 average over the past few years. The one thing that has always eluded me is the perfect 300 game. I have had many opportunities in the past when the shot was just right and I could string six or seven strikes to start a game, but my emotions would always get the best of me. I could never carry it all the way into the tenth frame. I should point out here that I took two years off from bowling and just picked it back up.

Last night, which was my first game in two years and also my first since learning EFT, was at first no different from any other night of bowling. I had a good 223 game to start and continued throwing strikes into the second game. The big difference last night was that when I got past the sixth strike, I started thinking about EFT. In between frames, I just sat in my chair tapping on the Karate Chop point and concentrating on staying calm.

This is the point in the game where my knees would normally turn to jelly and I would throw a bad shot. Not last night. I stayed calm all the way into the tenth frame. The first shot in the tenth crossed over "Brooklyn" and just carried the 10 pin. The second ball was good and I was only one strike away. I stood at the end of the approach and could see a bowler a couple lanes to my right, so I waited while he finished bowling.

All the while I tapped the Karate Chop point on my right hand against the ball return and concentrated on the final shot. I could feel a quiver go through me just as I positioned the ball for my last approach and I smoothly delivered the ball just as I had in the previous 11 shots. Everyone watching said it was my best shot of the night. It hit flush in the pocket and crushed everything except the 7 pin, which slowly leaned to the left and fell into the gutter for the elusive perfect game.

I finished the night with a 183 game to give me a 706 series, but I attribute the "300" game to EFT's ability to keep my emotions in check and allowing my body to do the rest.

❊ ❊ ❊

Here is a classic case where collapsing some limiting beliefs and doubts with EFT results in a stellar performance. The object of lawn bowling is to roll a ball, or bowl, closest to the target ball, a small white ball called a jack. The ball's design, which is slightly flattened on one side, creates the challenge of the game. Its shape causes the ball to travel a curved path, or bias. Prior to using EFT, Dorothy Goudie considered herself more of a background figure than a competitor in this sport. Not any more!

Dorothy refers to EFT's finger points, which are described in Appendix A.

An EFT Lawn Bowling Championship
by Dorothy Goudie

I had been reading about EFT for sports improvements and as our New Zealand lawn bowling club championships were to be contested, I decided to try some tapping. Ours is a small club but the competition is serious and titles are well defended. I would not say that I'm a competitive person—in fact, I don't play very much at all—but I enjoy the relaxation of it when I do. I explored all the ideas that I held about being a winner and beating others.

Even though I'm not an expert, don't bowl as much as other members do, and I feel guilty about beating someone I think is better than me, I deeply and completely accept myself.

Even though I feel bad about beating anyone and need to keep my place in the pecking order and not over-step my position…

Even though the green is too slow, the shot is too difficult for me, I can't do run shots, the wind is too strong, this shot is too difficult, the opposition is just too good, and I'm not good enough…

Even though winning is not that important to me so why am I trying to beat someone to whom it is important…

Then I went a step further:

Even though I'm scared that if I am champion I will have to compete on the next level, and then I'll be up against the big guns, I deeply and completely accept myself.

Even though people in the bowling world will notice me, what if I let myself down, I don't have the time to put in the practice needed to compete on that level…

Even though all these things are true, I choose to play to the best of my ability no matter who that competition is…it's OK to stand out…I will be steady and remember the basics and not be distracted by anything including the weather. I love and approve of myself, win or lose.

Then I recited the famous Marianne Williamson quote:

Even though my deepest fear is not that I am inadequate, my deepest fear is that I am powerful beyond measure…

And I ended with:

And as I let my own light shine I give others permission to do the same and I am liberated from my own fear.

During the game whenever I was feeling anxious, I mentally tapped or did rapid tapping on the finger points with my thumb, while mentally saying, "You can do it, keep to the basics, take your time and follow through."

The result was that I won every game I played by quite a margin and am now the club's Women's Singles Champion. People may say that it is just a coincidence and I would have won anyway, but I don't think so. Now I will go on and play in the Champion of Champions against the best from all the region's clubs and that will be the test. Isn't this tapping fun!

❀ ❀ ❀

Note how EFT newcomer Stefaunia Dhillon from the U.K. applies EFT to a novice golfer and dramatically improves his score from the mid-40s to 27 on a short nine-hole course. This is an improvement of approximately 40 percent, which is impressive by anyone's standards. It exceeds the golf achievement of my son, Adam, that appears onscreen in the EFT Course video. Adam went from an average of 55-60 to 43 in one day, also on a short nine-hole course.

40-percent Improvement, Golf Tournament Win

by Stefaunia Dhillon

My second attempt with EFT was at a golf course in Newbury, England. I met with a man who wanted to shoot in the low 30s. He had been shooting in the mid-40s on a nine-hole course.

The first time out with him we tapped for anxiety the first few rounds, but then he realized that if he could keep his head still he would make better shots.

So we tapped for "Head still, focus." Sure enough, by the end of the ninth hole he had scored 34. We dramatically improved his game.

He approached me several days later saying he wanted to improve that 34 by several more strokes. So I walked the course with him and by the ninth hole he had scored 27.

He than told me that he would be playing in three tournaments at an 18-hole golf course that weekend. He had never won before and was hoping he would do well.

That following Monday I received a phone call from him. He was on "cloud nine" because he broke the course record of 60 and won all three tournaments. He was very, very happy.

✿ ✿ ✿

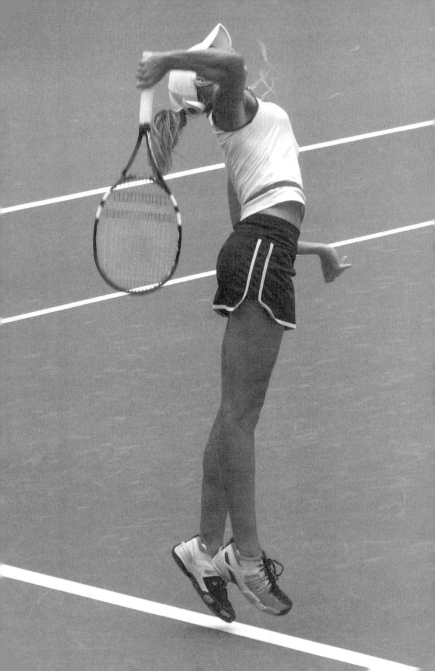

5

EFT for
Sports Injuries

Every sport has its signature injuries. Think of tennis elbow, runner's knee, Little League elbow, golfer's elbow, cycler's road rash, swimmer's ear, rower's shoulder syndrome, surfer's knot, and skier's thumb. Then you have baseball and football with their torn rotator cuff and cruciate ligament injuries; the frozen shoulder common in softball, tennis, swimming, and weight training; and all the pulled muscles, muscle cramps, shin splints, and sprains that can afflict any athlete.

While the rest of the world may go ho-hum at athletic injuries, professional sports teams take them quite seriously. They pay their athletes g'zillions of greenies and don't like it when their "investments" are sitting idle on the sidelines nursing various aches and pains. Do you suppose they might appreciate someone who could speed up the healing process for even 25 percent of these injuries? What about 50 percent? Or 75 percent?

Some of EFT's most dramatic success stories involve recovery from accidents and injuries. This brief article by Cathy Reid from Canada points up EFT's potential using the Basic Recipe all by itself. If the pain doesn't disappear, there are many EFT refinements you can apply, but the Basic Recipe is always worth trying first.

EFT Cures a Two-year Case of Tennis Elbow

by Cathy Reid

I am a Certified Personal Trainer, and for the past two years, I have had tennis elbow. It was so bad I couldn't even open a jar. I went for laser treatments, had massage therapy, and wore an arm brace, all with only temporary benefits. I love to lift heavy weights and could not do so because of severe arm pain. I read about EFT and started applying this by using the simple Setup Phrase:

Even though I have tennis elbow, I deeply and completely accept myself.

I tapped seven times on each of the EFT points while saying the Reminder Phrase *"tennis elbow."* I did this three or four times a day, and at the end of a week my level of intensity had gone from a 10 on the 0-to-10 scale down to zero. The pain is gone and I am lifting heavy weights once again. Thanks to EFT, I have my life back and I feel very strong again.

❊ ❊ ❊

We've already demonstrated that EFT can improve and enhance sports performance. Now physical and occupational therapists, chiropractors, massage therapists, coaches, trainers, and others who learn EFT have a head start in fixing injuries of every description. Listen in as seasoned EFT'er Roseanna Ellis easily and consistently provides benefits for university-caliber athletes. Someday professional sports teams will fall all over themselves to get these results.

An EFT Sports Injury Therapist's Morning
by Roseanna Ellis

I thought I would share my yesterday morning therapy at Monmouth University in New Jersey. I am a sports injury consultant for the top athletes at the University and have a contract with the school to provide treatment for those who can't get better through regular physical therapy or athletic training.

The first athlete came in with no complaints of any pain or tightness because he had seen me for a few visits and had 100 percent success on his hamstring injury, very tight hamstrings, and low back pain. But he was concerned about his athletic performance. His goal was to change a bad habit he had when throwing and he wanted to be able to leap up into the air to clear a bar.

We performed EFT on his throwing habit for 10 minutes; then we worked on his spring jump for 10 minutes. When he first jumped his hand was about six to eight inches from the ceiling. After 10 minutes of EFT his hand could easily reach the ceiling with no problem. I spent the last 10 minutes stretching him. He was very pleased.

Next came a young lady who performed Lacrosse. She had low back and hip pain which extended down the side of her leg. We worked on numerous issues such as pain at level 6 on the 0-to-10 intensity scale, fear of failure, and hip tightness. Within 20 minutes she was pain-free and felt very confident.

The third was a young lady who played softball. She was very concerned because she had played two games the day before and was scheduled for two more that afternoon and evening. She had severe knee pain measuring 8 on the right, 6 on the left, and 10 when using stairs. She also had a fear of failing. I worked for about five minutes on her knee caps to decrease any adhesions. Then we performed EFT on the pain until it came down to zero while walking. We worked for another 10 minutes on stair climbing until she was able to step up without pain. A normal step is about 8 inches, and she could step up a 12-inch step without pain or discomfort. Then we did EFT for five minutes on her fear.

The fourth was a male athlete who injured his left hamstring while running. His pain was 8 to 9. His hamstrings were very tight. For an athlete, this means trouble, not only because it puts him at a higher risk of injury but it weighs him down so much that his agility is compromised greatly.

I worked on his pain with EFT for about 20 minutes until it came down to zero (this took longer than usual because he had never seen such weird therapy). Then with 10 minutes of Active Isolated Stretching he gained 25 to 30 degrees of motion – full range and then some. He was blown out of the water.

You can see how much can be accomplished in the 30 minutes that I have with each of these athletes. Thanks to EFT, days like this happen all the time.

✿ ✿ ✿

Sam Smith writes from Australia about the leg and back cramping he experienced while playing soccer – and the relief that a few minutes of EFT produced. Note that Sam's results from that single tapping session have lasted for months.

Soccer and Leg Cramps

by Sam Smith

I've been using EFT with work colleagues for a variety of problems. One girl had a phobia of elevators but now happily uses the one in our building. The same girl has gone from at least a packet of cigarettes a day to maybe one or two. She feels "settled" with this amount and I haven't pushed it further. EFT has been successful on a variety of issues and I'm learning all the time.

I'm 44 and have been a fanatic soccer player all my life. But these past three years or so I've been suffering from cramp. Mostly it would be in the legs and feet but occasionally in the lower back. It was normally as I lay in bed at night and it could really disrupt my rest as well as being quite painful. I could always feel its onset but no matter what I did I couldn't shake it off. It could be excruciating. Until EFT, that is.

I was experiencing cramp in my leg one night when my wife suggested that I try EFT. I just hadn't thought about it. It took three rounds to get it down to a 1 on the 0-to-10 scale. Then another two rounds to make it disappear. I was ecstatic. But get this. That was nearly three months ago and I've experienced cramp only once since the original treatment. That was last week and it required only two rounds of EFT to get it to go away. And this from a guy who was *suffering from cramp at least three to four times per week!* Brilliant!!!

❄ ❄ ❄

In this next report, Sejual Shah from the U.K. uses some very creative approaches to eliminate an athlete's long-standing knee pain. In this case, each of his knees had a different story to tell.

EFT for Knee Pain

by Sejual Shah

Paul is a keen cyclist who competes in triathalons. Any improvements, large or small, would help him improve his game. As we used EFT to treat his pain, we discovered that by taking each knee separately, each had a different story to tell.

Paul's problems with his knees date back more than 20 years. The constant soreness in his left knee could be traced to when he was 21 and playing football (soccer). He ran past a player who tried to tackle him and the knee just collapsed inward, on itself. The knee was bruised and very painful. Ever since that event, his left knee felt constantly rough and stiff. During the 20 years since the soccer incident, no physiotherapist or chiropractor could eliminate the pain. When we started tapping, the pain was at a 4 on the 0-to-10 scale.

Even though it feels like I've got a spongy "doughnut" behind my left knee, I deeply and completely accept myself.

Even though I hurt it so badly whilst playing football when I was 21…

Even though I thought it wasn't a problem at the time…

Even though my knee was black and blue from the tackle, and it still remembers that bruising experience to this day…

Paul reported feeling odd sensations in his left knee, as if something was moving around inside. I asked him to tell me more about what happened when he was 21. It was an away match and he was sharing a hotel room with other team members. After the match he was in a huge amount of constant pain. Later that evening he couldn't fall asleep. He remembered hearing the easy sleep of his team members and feeling frustrated and panic-stricken.

Even though it feels like I've got John Hurt in my knee, I deeply and completely accept myself.

Humor's great for helping ease any concerns someone is feeling about odd temporary sensations in the body.

Even though I was in excruciating pain, and they didn't care…

Even though I couldn't think of anything but my poor knee and what would happen to it…

Even though I was angry that my teammates were enjoying an easy sleep and not suffering like I was…

Even though I was deeply worried about what would happen to my knee in the future…

Astonished, he discovered that there was no tension left in his knee. It felt fine when walking in my treatment room. A week later he reported there had been a tremendous improvement in the knee, and the pain was virtually at a zero. He was happy with it.

The following week we decided to tackle the right knee, which had a different story to tell. Paul was diagnosed four years ago with his right leg being shorter than his left. Given his huge enjoyment of sports, this had an impact on his hips and spine and the rest of his body. His joints had to compensate for the defect and were stretched beyond the normal 20 percent they could naturally cope with.

He had custom insoles for his shoes made four years ago and since then his body was properly aligned. However, his right knee hadn't improved and on the 0-to-10 scale he'd get a 2-level pain if he pushed it. He felt discomfort particularly when running downhill, when he had to shift his weight onto the balls of his feet to maintain balance.

We tapped on the following:

Even though my right knee hasn't caught up with mechanical changes I've made to support it and my body, I deeply and completely accept myself.

Even though my right knee is worried that things will go bad again and it has to hold out just in case…..

Even though my right knee is scared of losing control and afraid that I'll tumble down because I'm not balanced…

Even though I need to be in control to avoid harming myself, I instead choose to feel I'm always in balance…

Paul nodded with understanding as each Setup was delivered—he could see where I was going and it felt right. I checked in with him between each round and at the end Paul noted he'd felt a shift in his knee. In particular, he appreciated the subtle change we were introducing by replacing "control" with "balance." He realized his performance could be effortless. During the session he tested his knee by walking down stairs and noticed a definite improvement.

It's now eight weeks later. Our work on his right knee has held and he has no problems that stop him from running.

Paul and I worked on several other sports performance issues, such as maintaining motivation. He explained how in previous years he always felt emotionally down in February and March as other demands on his time would mean that he couldn't do a long cycle ride of 50 miles plus. This year, however, as a result of our work he felt calm when the situation arose yet again. Instead of feeling depressed, he was making plans to fit a long ride in whenever possible and was no longer beating himself up about the situation.

Overall, Paul's levels of self-appreciation improved, and he noticed subtle benefits on top of the mechanical improvements we achieved for his knees.

Here's what he said recently about our work: "I'm a logical person with a scientific background and so was skeptical when Sejual offered EFT for a minor ailment, a runny nose that had been around for several weeks. I was very surprised when a few minutes of tapping eradicated my snuffles. Since then we've worked on my motivation to train for triathlon competitions and knee problems from old injuries. During eight sessions we tapped on related issues. My commitment to train has significantly improved. My confidence in tackling a very challenging part of the Tours de Flanders cycle race has rocketed up. The soreness I have had in both knees for more 20 years has simply melted away. My running is much smoother than before the tapping. I'd recommend EFT to other athletes for any physical and mental blocks that are holding them back from achieving their goals."

❊ ❊ ❊

Ron Ball's wife injured her shoulder and a local doctor thought she had a torn rotator cuff that might require surgery. Some simple rounds of EFT brought rapid relief and, the next day, the problem was nowhere to be found.

Rapid Relief for a Torn Rotator Cuff

by Ron Ball

EFT can be a surprisingly good healing tool regarding accidents. Recently, my wife went grocery shopping. She used a smaller, different cart than she normally does. On her way to the car with her groceries, she tripped over the cart and fell. She was scuffed up, in pain, and had limited motion in her left arm.

When she got home, she spoke to my neighbor about it. A talented and compassionate doctor, he said that most likely she had a torn rotator cuff and that it might require surgery. Since I recommend trying EFT on everything, that afternoon we did a few rounds of tapping.

Here are some of the setup phrases we used:

Even though I felt awkward when I tripped over the grocery cart, I deeply and completely accept myself.

Even though it surprised and really scared me, I deeply and completely accept myself.

Even though I took a bad fall, I deeply and completely accept myself.

We were open to the idea that EFT might or might not help. After all, we were dealing with a "physical problem." It was pretty amazing. After a few rounds of EFT, the pain diminished and her arm's range of motion increased dramatically. What's even more interesting is that the next day, it was as if she'd forgotten there was ever an issue with her arm. There has been no problem since.

In my opinion, what many doctors and healthcare professionals miss is that they need to address the stress, emotional trauma, and shock to the system when a person trips over a cart, falls off a ladder, or gets hurt in a minor accident. In addition to real physical issues, there could be embarrassment, shame, or any number of emotional factors. What might have happened with my wife's arm if she hadn't been open the idea of trying EFT on everything?

※ ※ ※

Physicians, sports doctors, and anyone associated with athletic injuries will enjoy this "impossible" result from Gillian Tarawhiti of Australia.

Rapid Results for an ACL Tear

by Gillian Tarawhiti

I was injured in a sports accident incurring an anterior cruciate ligament (ACL) injury and a meniscus cartilage tear. Basically this means I had ligament and cartilage tears in my knee. I was immediately referred to specialists, had an MRI, and was told I would need major surgery and that I would have difficulty with my knee for the rest of my life.

Well, I'm an EFT practitioner and decided to take their diagnosis with a grain of salt. I decided to postpone any surgery against the advice of my specialist and surgeons. I decided to take my own journey and tapped religiously for everything from pain to feeling stupid for letting it happen, to over-stretching, to blaming everyone else, and on and on. Five days after I started tapping I was back doing some light training. Two weeks after that I was doing even more training even though everyone tried to tell me that is was not a good idea and that I should slow down or not train at all. But you know, I was feeling good, I still obviously had an injury but I knew my limits and continued to tap and train anyway.

Last week I went for a second MRI. When I saw my specialist, he couldn't believe that the ACL tears had disappeared. He kept going back and forth between the first and second MRI images and couldn't believe it. He said he had never in his entire career see an injury like the one I had incurred just disappear. It made me laugh that he refused to say "fix itself." But there it was on his screen in the before-and-after images.

When he asked what I had done in the past four months, I told him I went back to training straight away and that I was doing a form of physiotherapy. I knew he had to ask what it was, so I explained in as much technical terminology as I could muster about

Emotional Freedom Techniques. He stared at me for a moment and said, "Well, you will do me out of a job if anyone else finds out about this." We both laughed and then he looked at me and said, "No! I'm not joking."

I am so grateful that my injury now is minor and requires only microscopic day surgery to which I've agreed since there will be no slicing or dicing. So all you sports people out there—EFT works, it really does.

❊ ❊ ❊

In this next example, Dr. John Ford of Nova Scotia, Canada, describes how his inexperienced client applied EFT to himself for a sprained ankle. Instead of taking the week or two one would normally expect, his recovery was almost immediate.

EFT Ankle Sprain Recovery

by John Ford, N.D.

I have been doing EFT for just over two years and have had great success both for myself and clients.

Bill, a friend of mine, telephoned me Saturday morning to say that he had to change some plans we had made for Sunday because he had sprained his ankle. The swelling was immediate and severe.

When I was talking with him his ankle was severely swollen and he described the pain as throbbing. He needed crutches to get around and expected that he would be off work for at least a few days.

I had introduced EFT to Bill a few months earlier and thus suggested that he tap for the swelling and pain in his ankle. I did not actually work with him on the phone but instead gave him EFT instructions to do on his own. I simply advised him to tap on the EFT points and at the same time focus on the pain that he was experiencing. He assured me that he would not have a problem with the latter.

He tapped again a few times Saturday afternoon and evening for the swelling and pain. When he woke up Sunday morning and put his feet to the floor he realized that there was no throbbing in his ankle. Furthermore, there was no swelling. Later that day he went to a hockey game and had to walk three blocks from where he parked his car to the arena and back. However, there was no swelling or pain in his ankle.

On Monday morning Bill called me at 8:00 AM. He was at work. In fact, he had driven there on his motorcycle. He then explained that, when he woke up, his crutches were beside the bed so he thought he would use them to stand up. While sitting on the edge of the bed he started to bend his foot and ankle and realized that he could do so without pain. Except for some minor stiffness (which disappeared after he stretched his ankle) he was able to get up and walk around, without the crutches, totally pain-free. No swelling. No pain. No discoloration.

I asked him if he could explain the quick recovery and he said, "It had to be the tapping because I didn't do anything else."

❀ ❀ ❀

Stacey Vornbrock, an EFT sports performance expert in Scottsdale, Arizona, has carved out a growing niche for herself in the sports world. On page 137, she discussed EFT and sports statistics. Here she shows how EFT helps athletes improve their kicking, swinging, and other important movements. After rapidly improving a batting swing, Stacey says, *"It would normally take hundreds of swings to achieve a similar result."*

EFT and Mechanical Improvements

by Stacey Vornbrock

I have been using EFT to help professional and amateur athletes make mechanical changes since 2003. It's an easy and fast way for these guys to get results that would normally take months or even years to accomplish.

Whenever you attempt to make a mechanical change, you're fighting against a habit that is literally held in every cell membrane of your body. Every time your body makes the new movement, your cells fight to re-establish the old pattern. Change feels difficult and uncomfortable because you're not only fighting the habit that is trying to re-establish itself but you're also directing your body to move in ways it isn't used to or comfortable with. With EFT it's easy to give your body the instruction to release the old habit and adapt to the new movement.

All I need to know is what an athlete is currently doing that is causing a problem and what he or she would rather be doing. One of the first questions I ask is, "What are you afraid will happen if you do it the way you want to do it?" I've discovered that frequently, but not always, there is a fear of an unwanted result that drives athletes to make the mechanical movement they're currently making. Let me give you some examples.

"Robert" is a talented college football kicker destined for the National Football League next year. Mechanically his issue was bringing his right leg across his body when he kicks. He was afraid that if he kicked with his leg straighter, he would hook the ball left or punch it right. Here are the things we tapped on.

Even though I'm holding this habit of bringing my leg across my body when I kick in every cell of my body, I deeply and completely accept myself.

Then we used a different Reminder Phrase on each tapping point, such as:

I can't kick straight. I'm afraid I'll hook it left or punch it right. I don't have the velocity I need. I don't have the power I need. It feels so uncomfortable when I keep my leg straight. I played soccer all those years and my body is used to bringing my leg across. I feel like I'm doing something wrong when I keep my leg straight. It feels unnatural to keep my leg straight through the kick.

New Setup Phrases included:

Even though this habit of bringing my leg across my body is locked in every cell of my right leg, I deeply and completely accept myself.

Even though when I get anxious, my body reverts to this old habit of kicking across my body, I deeply and completely accept myself.

These were followed by new Reminder Phrases:

I'm holding this habit of bringing my right leg across my body in all the muscles of my right leg. I'm holding this habit of bringing my right leg across my body in all the ligaments of my right leg. I'm holding this habit of bringing my right leg across my body in all the tendons of my right leg. I'm holding this habit of bringing my right leg across my body in all the bones of my right leg. I'm holding this habit of bringing my right leg across my body in all the joints of my right leg. I'm holding this habit of bringing my right leg across my body in all the cartilage of my right leg. I'm holding this habit of bringing my right leg across my body in all the tissues of my right leg. I'm holding this habit of bringing my right leg across my body in all the nerves of my right leg. I'm holding this habit of bringing my right leg across my body in all the fascia of my right leg. I'm holding this habit of bringing my right leg across my body in all the membranes of my right leg. I'm holding this habit of bringing my right leg across my body in all the skin of my right leg. I'm holding this habit of bringing my right leg across my body in all the fluids of my right leg. I'm holding this habit of bringing my right leg across my body in all the fibers of my right leg.

I've found that it makes a significant difference if you tap on the habit residing in the body. The body responds by releasing the habit much faster this way. Robert and I tapped for this problem only once and that took care of it.

Here are two mechanical examples involving "John," a Major League Baseball player. The first issue for him was that he was using his arms and shoulders to swing the bat rather than using his lats (the latissimus dorsi muscle in his middle back). His fear was that he would lose his eye/hand coordination if he were to swing using his lats. Here's what we tapped on:

Even though I'm not using my lats to swing, I'm relying on my arms and shoulders and it doesn't come natural to me to use my lats, I deeply and completely accept myself.

We used a different Reminder Phrase at each tapping point:

I don't remember to use my lats. It feels comfortable to use my arms. It feels safer to use my arms and shoulders. I'm not exploding from my upper legs. I'm afraid to get my legs involved. My upper body and lower body aren't working together. I only pay attention to my upper body and my eyes. I'll lose my eye/hand coordination if I use my lats to swing. I won't make solid contact with the ball if I use my lats. My body is in the habit of swinging and moving with my upper body only.

After tapping on this issue just one time, John was able to swing using his lats and explode from his legs. It felt natural and easy for him as if he'd always been doing this. A change like this would normally take hundreds of practice swings to achieve.

I tap with all my professional baseball players for seeing the ball sooner when it leaves the pitcher's hand. After tapping on this issue, players report that the game slows down for them, the ball appears big and bright to them, and they can pick up the ball at the release point. We tap on fastballs, sliders or curve balls, and change-ups. Here's how John and I tapped for fastballs:

Even though I can't see the ball release from the pitcher's hand, I only see it when it's on me, I deeply and completely accept myself.

Even though the ball looks so dark and I can't see the seams when they're end-over-end, I deeply and completely accept myself.

The Reminder Phrases included:

I can't see the ball. The ball looks so dark. My eyes can't pick up the seams. My brain can't register the direction of the seams fast enough My eyes and brain aren't in harmony with seeing the fastball. I can't slow the ball down. Nothing is in slow motion. The ball looks so small. My mind is not in harmony with the fastball. My body timing isn't in harmony with hitting the ball. I'm out of sync with responding to the ball. My head moves and everything jumps. When I'm jumpy the ball appears smaller. I feel so anxious when the ball appears small.

"Stan" is a Gateway Tour golfer. He was working on a small mechanical change in his golf swing with his teaching pro but he was struggling to get this last little piece in place. His fear was that the club would get too far behind him and he would lose control during the swing. Here's what we tapped on:

Even though I can't take the club back with my right side and I push down with my thumb and shove it back, I deeply and completely accept myself.

Even though I squeeze with my right thumb and can't relax my right thumb, I deeply and completely accept myself.

We tapped the EFT points with these Reminder Phrases:

I can't take the club back. I push down with my thumb. I shove it back. I squeeze with my right thumb. I can't relax my right thumb. It's such a habit to push with my right thumb and index finger. I'm still trying to keep from getting the club behind me. I especially do this when I feel pressure or a tough shot. I'm trying to control the shot and this is how I do it. I'm afraid the club will get too far behind me. I'll end up coming over the top.

We tapped on this only once and he was able to make the change he wanted easily and comfortably. The standard thinking in the world of golf is that it can take up to a year to change a swing. Thankfully that's no longer true with EFT!

❈ ❈ ❈

Here is another fascinating report from Stacey regarding her athletic clients' all-important range of motion. This is a "must read" for anyone in the performance field.

Range of Motion and Sports Performance

by Stacey Vornbrock

I first used EFT with range of motion (ROM) issues in 2003 when I started working with a golfer who was a Nationwide Tour Player. When I met him, his hip flexors were so tight that he couldn't rotate fully around into his back swing. In order to get around, he was lifting his left foot off the ground, a big no-no as this causes instability and a host of other problems.

His golf pro asked if I could do something about his tight hip flexors. I said, "Sure, let's try it, it won't make things worse!"

Within two rounds of tapping, he was able to keep his left foot rock-solid on the ground and his hip rotation increased from about 20 to 40 degrees. His golf pro was speechless.

The next day his golf pro was stretching him on the table when I arrived and he told me we had 40-degree rotation but still needed another 5 degrees. I said, "No problem," and we started tapping. In front of our eyes his hip rotated another 10 degrees. When I learned that this golfer had experienced a pretty traumatic left hip injury, we tapped on all aspects of that injury.

The golf pro and I were very excited by this and I started experimenting with other golfers, all with great results, but with no specific measurable proof.

Then in September of 2004, a local company contacted me because they were interested in the work I do with athletes. They use sensors and a very high-tech program to measure golf and baseball swings and motion of every kind.

I met with their athletic trainer, Marilyn, who gave me three people and provided verifiable measurements of their range of motion before and after EFT.

The first client was John, an athlete in his mid-thirties who had been in a car accident about two months prior. He had injured his neck and shoulders. Marilyn had been working with him for one month with no results.

At the end of our first session John had an increase in ROM of 67 percent, and by the end of our second session his symptoms were gone. (Remember, Marilyn had worked for a month with him with no results.)

I explained to her that whenever there is an injury or surgery, there are three major areas to address on the cellular level.

The first is the trauma to the body itself. That trauma immediately settles into the cell receptors around the injury and will just stay there unless you signal the cell receptors to release it. Along with trauma immediately come adrenaline, pain, and fear. Just because you aren't in pain or you don't feel any fear or adrenaline right now doesn't mean it has cleared out of your cell receptors. It's still sitting there and must be tapped on for maximum results.

The second area has to do with all the negative emotions you experience as a result of the injury. I call it the "oh damn" moment, where you realize what you've done and there is a cascade of thoughts and feelings about what this means to you, as well as any negative emotions around the rehab process. Anger, fear, frustration, embarrassment, weakness, loss of confidence, and fear of re-injury are common emotions that get stuck in the cell receptors around the injury site. It's critical to tap on all of the emotions to release them from the cell receptors because once released, those freed-up cell receptors are fully available to take in nutrients, proteins, vitamins, and minerals. All the things you're doing to heal (such as chiropractic care, nutritional supplements, physiotherapy, and massage) can then work at the deepest cellular level in your body.

Finally, whenever you are injured, the body immediately forms a memory of protection on the cellular level to keep that part of the body safe. You begin to hold yourself in a certain way and the body begins to adapt around the injury. Once the injury heals, nothing signals the body to release the memory of protection. Your body never returns to a state of balance but remains in that adaptive state. You will consciously or unconsciously hold back in the way you move your body, preventing you from performing at your highest level.

I have discovered that old injuries never fully heal because the trauma, emotions, and memory of protection have never been released from the cell receptor sites. Once the old trauma, emotions, and memory of protection are released, you may recover range of motion and be able to move your body in ways you haven't been able to for years, thus improving your athletic performance.

Our second client was Aaron, a 15-year-old baseball player. Marilyn was stretching his hamstrings and he was wincing. He had no injuries, just very tight hamstrings.

It had taken Marilyn two months to obtain a 20-degree range of motion in his hamstrings. In 30 seconds I was able to increase his range of motion from 20 to 45 degrees, which is more than a 200-percent increase. She was speechless!

The third client was Julie, a 16-year-old who plays softball and baseball. She had torn her anterior cruciate ligament (ACL), the ligament that helps hold the knee together, and she had surgery for that.

Julie missed a critical week of rehabilitation after the surgery, and months later she couldn't straighten her knee in order do the exercises that would strengthen muscles that hold the knee in place. Marilyn had worked with Julie for two months with no results. She was ready to recommend surgery to remove scar tissue deep in the knee.

By the end of our first session, we had 5 degrees range of motion and by the end of the second session, we had 20 degrees. This was enough for Julie to go home and start doing her exercises to strengthen her knee. This young woman was saved from having unnecessary surgery.

In 2005 I worked with Tom, a Major League Baseball pitcher, who had been out on the Disabled List for months. He had a torn ligament in his left shoulder from throwing. He came to see me to work on confidence issues related to pitching.

In the course of our work together, he decided to have surgery on his shoulder after an alternative treatment failed to produce the results he was looking for. Before the surgery, we tapped on issues such as his worry, doubt, and fear abound rehabbing his shoulder. I wanted to make sure that he went into surgery without any negative emotions sitting in his cells.

His surgery went very well and in fact the surgeon repaired two tears in his ligament. We had a session soon after his operation and we tapped for trauma, pain, fear, his body not being in harmony with the screws that had been inserted into his shoulder, the anesthesia, doubt that he would recover his range of motion, scar tissue, and memory of protection.

At his first rehab session, he could reach his left arm completely across his chest. His physical therapist said, "I don't understand this. I've never seen anything like this." The therapist explained that it would normally take four weeks for someone to achieve what Tom was doing on his first day of rehab.

It normally takes 16 weeks to recover from this surgery and we had already cut that time by one-fourth! Approximately one month later, the physical therapist took range-of-motion measurements and said to Tom, "Some of your measurements are better than normal. I don't understand this."

Then the surgeon told Tom his range of motion was excellent and his recovery was ahead of schedule. He made a full and complete recovery.

A college baseball catcher I work with had full "Tommy John surgery" at the end of August 2008. In this procedure, a ligament in the medial elbow is replaced with a tendon from somewhere else in the body, often from the forearm, hamstring, knee, or foot. Recovery takes about one year for pitchers and about six months for position players. His recovery time was expected to be that of a pitcher.

Within four months of our tapping work, he had clearance from his doctor to begin throwing and increase his lifting. At one point in his rehab process, he had so much flexibility in his elbow that his physiotherapist got scared and had him go for an MRI to make sure he hadn't damaged it again! Of course his MRI came back completely clear and he fully healed considerably ahead of schedule.

Another client, a former LPGA Tour Player and current golf coach, had over 28 past injuries. Despite a surgery and numerous rehab attempts, these old injuries impeded her coaching and her very athletic day-to-day life. Through patience and persistence we tapped on all her injuries. She reported that our EFT work revolutionized her recovery and she is now able to fully participate in all her sports and coaching without pain or discomfort.

I have worked with hundreds of athletes and every one of them has been injured at least once, many multiple times. Using the EFT protocols I've developed for injuries, I can consistently reduce recovery time from an athlete's surgery by at least three to four weeks and usually restore full range of motion.

Recovery time for current injuries is dramatically lessened, although that varies according to the specific injury. All the athletes I've worked with who have current injuries have been able to return to play much sooner than expected. When we complete the healing of old injuries through tapping, athletes report that aches and pains they've had for years are completely gone and they are able to play at the same level they played at pre-injury.

I've discovered that if there isn't an injury or an emotion held where the body is limited in range of motion, I can just tap without saying anything and movement happens immediately. However, if there is no increase in range of motion, I assume there is some emotional or physical trauma held in the cells there.

My experience has been that EFT's improvements in range of motion are permanent. If a client loses ground it simply indicates that there is something (usually emotional) that I missed.

I would encourage all of you to start experimenting first with yourself to increase your range of motion and then experiment with family and friends. When you have your own amazing results, contact chiropractors, massage therapists, doctors, and physical therapists and introduce them to EFT!

❀ ❀ ❀

At first glance this use of EFT for Deborah Miller's minor pulled muscle may seem quite routine. After all, it is not exactly life-threatening and EFT has certainly provided benefits for much more serious problems. However, pulled muscles can take highly paid professional athletes out of a game and can often sideline them, or impair their performance, for two or three more games. That is very expensive. Under those circumstances, what is a good EFT'er worth?

EFT for a Strained Muscle

by Deborah Miller, Ph.D.

I had an experience of stretching a muscle after falling into a hole. I enjoy testing the possibilities of what can be released with EFT so I figured I'd see if doing some immediate tapping would ease the discomfort. It did.

I was walking along a different area of the woods from where I normally walk. Actually it was alongside a cornfield in the mountains (they grow corn on the mountainsides where I live in Mexico). I stepped forward and my whole left leg dropped into a hole that I couldn't see because it was covered with tall grass. Now the leg that went into the hole didn't hurt at all, but my right leg hurt because of the speed with which the muscles had to contract to compensate for the lack of ground under my left leg.

I pulled my leg out of the hole and realized it was fine. After taking a few steps I realized the muscles in the calf area of my right leg ached. It wasn't bad but felt like a light pull. I could walk even though it ached, but I knew that it was one of those aches that would cause more problems the day after than immediately. I tapped briefly for the ache and especially for feeling stupid that I hadn't seen the hole (which was impossible to see even when looking at it directly). The ache went away and I walked on.

Later that evening the muscles started to stiffen again. I sat down and did more tapping on the foolishness of my walking somewhere I was not familiar with and not taking the appropriate precautions. This cornfield was near the edge of a ravine. So I tapped on all versions of my silliness and carelessness. Then I tapped on the physical ache and pulled muscles. I followed with tapping in the concept of a quick repair and relaxation of the muscles. Within minutes the ache went away and I forgot all about my perceived lack of carelessness. The pain never came back and I feel completely fine.

❈ ❈ ❈

Kaye Bewley from the U.K. gives us this brief account of clearing up a shoulder injury that just wasn't supposed to go away. Nonetheless it did, and this caused her client to exclaim, *"Ten years I've lived with that awful thing. How is that possible?"*

In addition to EFT's shortcut Basic Recipe, Kaye used the 9 Gamut Procedure, which is explained in Appendix A.

Annoying Shoulder 'Clunk' Disappears with EFT

by Kaye Bewley

Anne asked me to help her with a problem she suffered from for ten years. She had fallen off a horse and landed on her left shoulder. Everyone thought she had broken it because she was in so much pain, but x-rays showed nothing. Since that date, her shoulder has had an annoying click, rather like a clock mechanism. It does this every time she moves it round in a circle, when swimming, climbing onto horses, or just raising her arms. "It's like a clunk," she said. And I heard it myself. It was a really nasty little sound and quite loud.

We rated it at a 10, then did a round of tapping on the Karate Chop point, saying:

Even though I have this clunk in my left shoulder, I deeply and completely accept myself.

We did two rounds of tapping, then she moved her arm round in a big circle. The clunk was still there, although only very faint. She was amazed and rated it at 5 but said she accepted that it wouldn't disappear entirely. "It was a ligament, after all." She's a trained nurse and, of course, knows the body inside out.

We went through another round and it was still a 5, so we went through the 9 Gamut Procedure. Anne circled her arm again and looked at me as shock registered all over her face. "I can't believe that!" was all she kept repeating. She circled her arm several times, but there was no sound and no annoying feeling of a clunk. She kept trying to find it. I didn't want her to hurt herself so asked her to calm down with the circling, but she was too amazed. There was one tiny clunk, more of a minor "click," but that was all. She was totally amazed and pleased.

She said, "Ten years I've lived with that awful thing. How is that possible?"

Anne's rapid results may have startled her, but they were far from unusual in the world of EFT. I only wish I'd had Anne's shoulder clunk on video. If ever I had any doubts about EFT, they were squashed in those ten minutes!

※ ※ ※

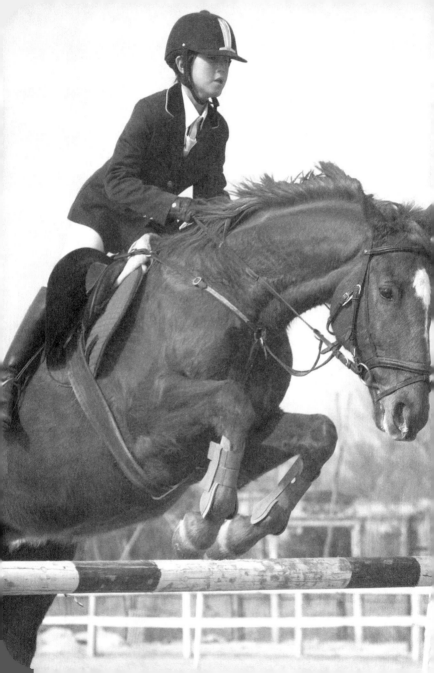

6

You're Never Too
Young or Too Old

That's true! No matter what your age, physical condition, training, or experience level, EFT can improve everything from your coordination and stamina to your final score.

One simple way to energize your workouts and feel better all over is to add EFT's Constricted Breathing Technique to your daily routine. This simple combination of EFT tapping and deep breathing was described on page 59. Here Paul Zelizer cleverly uses the technique for improved strength and fitness.

EFT Breathing Technique for Improved Fitness
by Paul Zelizer

We can live for days without water and weeks without food. However, without oxygen we die within minutes. Abundant oxygen is one of our most important needs. Yet, in the stress of modern life, our breathing often becomes restricted. This impacts all aspects of our health and well-being.

As a lifelong athlete and someone who specializes in using EFT for physical issues, I am well aware of the impact of stress on breathing. For the past two months, I've been using EFT's Constricted Breathing Technique to supercharge my daily workout. It's been very successful.

Here's what I do. At the start of each workout, I use the Constricted Breathing Technique to ensure that I am breathing in a relaxed and efficient way. It takes about 30 to 45 seconds. Then at least twice during the day and just before going to sleep I do the same.

For such a small investment of time, the results have been remarkable. My fitness routine combines martial arts, dance, bodybuilding, and bodyweight conditioning. I find that I have more energy, my workouts are crisper, and I'm recovering faster. I've lost fat and gained about 4 pounds of pure muscle.

A friend is fond of quoting Arnold Schwarzenegger as saying, "One lift with the breath is worth ten without." Taking these few moments in my day to make sure my breathing is optimal is having big results in my fitness level. In fact, just this morning when I gave a friend a hug, she exclaimed, "You seem really strong!"

❊ ❊ ❊

We don't promote EFT as a Fountain of Youth—but maybe we should. This is because people often gain renewed energy with EFT and this increased vitality often lasts well into the future. In this report, 71-year-old Richard Avon from the U.K. used EFT to improve his energy while playing squash. He says, *"What is still amazing me is that I became an entirely different person with the most enormous energy and speed."*

71-year-old Plays Squash with Youthful Energy

by Richard Avon

I learned EFT as part of a Bio-Energetic Medicine course. I really thought all this tapping was complete mumbo jumbo until the day after the final session.

When we did the tapping in pairs on Saturday, I said, "The thing that really bugs me is that I play squash with my friend, who is 15 years younger than I am, and I have only ever beat him in the match once, and that was on a day when he had something on his mind and wasn't feeling himself."

My partner tapped with me while saying,

Even though I always lose the match, I deeply and completely accept myself.

Then I remembered reading about Anthony Robbins working with Andre Agassi when Agassi was in a slump. Robbins asked him what he was thinking at the start of a match and Agassi replied that he was remembering the last time he played this opponent and what went wrong. Robbins said, "No! When you walk on court, just remember winning at Wimbledon." This resurrected Agassi's career.

So when we tapped next, I concluded by saying, *"Remember winning. Remember winning."*

That morning I walked on court at 9:45 having tapped before I left home.

At my age (71) I usually play the old bull strolling around slowly lobbing into the corners and trying to out-think Chris, who hits the ball hard. The first game took 15 minutes and I won it 9 to 4. But what astonished me apart from my mental focus was that I was playing like a 25-year-old with enormous energy and speed—like a tiger! It didn't matter where he put the ball, I got there.

The next game he got over the shock and really put on the pressure and I lost 5 to 9. (I thought, "Here we go!") In the third game I was trailing all the way but managed to equalize at 8 - 8. Chris won 10 - 8.

The fourth game came and Chris raced to 6 - 0, then I got two points so I was losing 2 - 7. I started to surreptitiously tap between each point and clawed back to a 7 - 7 tie.

Chris got the next point 8 - 7. Match point!

I tapped some more and tied the game at 8 - 8, then finally won it with a score of 10 - 8. Two games all.

I went to the loo (restroom) and did a thorough tap, ending with my positive Reminder Phrase, *"Remember winning. Remember winning."*

I won the decider 9 - 5. WOW! 3 - 2 to me! The match had taken 50 minutes for five games. Not for one moment did I think of anything but the next point! Again WOW!

Chris said afterwards, "What f*****g pills are you on? I've never seen you like this." I just smiled graciously!

What is still amazing me is that I became an entirely different person with the most enormous energy and speed. If I were to compare the improvement to my normal play on the 0-to-10 scale, I would give this a 25!

I am now 74 and have beaten Chris on many occasions since then, using my surreptitious tapping. Strangely, I have never told him how I do it!!

❊ ❊ ❊

Coaches and parents who teach their kids how to use EFT give them a wonderful gift, one that will last a lifetime. Here are two short reports from EFT practitioner Denise Wall showing how the technique helped two young athletes overcome their fears and negative self-talk.

Sports EFT for Children

by Denise Wall

Jane is nine years old. She has been studying gymnastics for six years and is a star in her gym. She suddenly became fearful and refused to return to practice.

The interview revealed that she was learning to do a handstand backwards on the balance beam, and she was afraid that her hands did not know what to do, the problem being that she didn't know how to fall if she had to. We tapped on her fear of falling, not knowing how to fall, fear of being hurt, fear of having people watch her fall, and fear of letting her team down. Then, after the tapping, I asked her to see herself moving backward on the beam, see herself knowing how to fall, knowing where her hands could go, how her knees could bend, how she could land and re-mount. She mentally practiced falling skillfully and re-mounting. She practiced having her hands know where to go. She practiced her feet landing on the sweet spot of the beam.

The problem was gone. I asked her mom to have her review falling safely with her coach and to walk it through on the grounded balance beam. Jane returned to her gym and moved up to the next level. I met her mom several months later and she said that only one other time did they need to tap and Jane has been fine ever since.

Paul, who is 13, plays basketball. In practice, he can make 28 out of 30 baskets. In the basketball game, however, he falls apart. We tapped on falling apart and discovered that "I am too slow" had become his negative self-talk.

We tapped on being slow. The self-talk was the driver. I had him imagine making good shots that rose from the belly button, then rolled through his torso and out his fingertips. Now when he imagined the next game, he said he felt more relaxed than ever.

❊ ❊ ❊

In the next report, Shannon Hendrix applies EFT in two areas of her 12-year-old son's life, both with remarkable success. At one point Shannon has her son use the 9 Gamut Procedure, which is explained in Appendix A.

Better Soccer and Fast Recovery from Surgery

by Shannon Hendrix

I have had two remarkable successes in the past few days regarding my 12-year-old son, Wes. The first is in regard to his sports skills, and the second deals with a swift recovery from oral surgery just two days later.

I had tried EFT with my son and his friend on the way to a soccer game several months ago. I attempted to use the traditional Setup Phrase, "Even though I have this problem…" but it didn't quite work with two overconfident adolescents! After their team lost the game and they had no individual accomplishments from that particular game, they both gave me the "See, it didn't work, Mom" attitude.

However, recently my son was up at 6 AM preparing for a tournament. He candidly spoke to me about his nerves and fears that he would "forget" the things he had been trained to do once he got on the field. The members of this team hadn't practiced together because they were combined from separate teams.

He allowed me to quietly tap several points while he talked about the negative situations he was mentally picturing. He is usually quite confident and doesn't often admit insecurities in this way. I didn't use an "I'm still a really great kid" ending; I just tapped while he spoke his concerns.

That evening, he came home with a medal. His team had won the entire tournament and he had five goals (more than he had scored all season), two of which were spectacular crowd-pleasers, as well as several assists!

Two days later, Wes had an appointment with the oral surgeon to have four molars pulled for orthodontic reasons. He woke up nervous about the intravenous anesthesia and uncomfortable about not being able to eat for six hours before the mid-day surgery.

He wouldn't let me tap on him before surgery, but as he came out of anesthesia, I tapped him gently as I spoke to him, encouraging him to wake him up as the nurse had directed me to do. He didn't fight or bat my hand away and I only spoke "waking up, eyes are blinking" type statements aloud.

I continued to tap as it seemed appropriate over the next several minutes, not every point, and not always speaking out loud, but I had thoughts of controlling the bleeding and of course, the pain that was sure to come after numbness wore off. I did direct him to roll his eyes, hum, and count as I tapped the Gamut point, to which he obediently complied, though groggy.

After bringing him home to my husband, I returned to work for several hours. Imagine my surprise and delight upon my return a few hours later to see him up and around, eating comfortably, chatting cheerfully, and speaking of being sore, not numb, and with no trace of pain at all.

He took only one dose of pain medication and actually asked to go to school the next day, even though it would have been an excused absence through two more days. He has little or no noticeable swelling (which I didn't even think to tap for) and only iced his jaw for a few minutes instead of 24 hours as directed. I am stunned, amazed, and thrilled at how my novice effort has paid off big time for my son in these two keenly important areas in his world!

※ ※ ※

When it comes to EFT, kids are naturals. They may, out of feelings of self-consciousness, resist at first, but as soon as they see it in action, they catch on fast. Here's a short report of how Val Piacitelli helped her young son. Val refers to the tender spot (also called the Sore Spot), which is on the chest. It can be massaged as an alternative to Karate Chop tapping. See Appendix A for details.

Bowling Performance and EFT

by Val Piacitelli

My eight-year-old son Benjamin was very discouraged when he went bowling. His scores were low and he was about to give up. I gently took him aside and asked him if he wanted to knock down all the pins in one shot. "Of course!," he said. With that, I had him rub his tender spot and recite,

> *Even though I am just learning to bowl, I deeply and completely accept myself.*

Even I was amazed when Ben's six-pound ball knocked over all ten pins immediately after his statements were said. He jumped for joy and gave me a memorable hug that nearly knocked me over, too!

EFT to me means *Ending Fearful Thoughts*. Spread this wonderfully contagious healing message like wildfire to children. After all, they are our future.

❁ ❁ ❁

It always delights me when someone with little or no experience does well in a sport, especially if EFT helps that happen. Arden Compton used EFT and blew the doors off of his previous bowling scores.

Novice Bowler Gets Eight Strikes in a Row

by Arden Compton

Recently I took my family bowling. The bowling alley here in Brigham City was giving away a turkey to anyone who bowled three strikes in a row. So, off we went to try our luck.

Now, I am not a serious bowler. Throughout my life, I have probably gone bowling about once a year…maybe less. I usually bowl somewhere between 100 and 120. If I get over 120, it is a good game for me. If I score above 130, that's a really good game. So, getting three strikes in a row wasn't likely. I might get two or three strikes in a game, but not in a row.

In my first frame, I knocked over eight pins, not bad. But I thought about how much fun it would be to win a turkey and I decided to try some EFT.

Even though I'm afraid of not making a strike, I deeply and completely accept myself.

On my next turn, as I held the ball in my right hand, I tapped with my left hand on the face points and repeated in my mind the Reminder Phrase, *This fear of not making a strike.*

It took a little over five seconds to tap through that. This time I bowled a spare (meaning I knocked all the pins over in two tries), but was only one pin away from getting a strike. Each turn for the rest of the game, I went through the same tapping process. The next frame I bowled a strike! But on my next turn's two frames I bowled a spare. I needed three strikes in a row.

I was feeling pretty good about my game at this point because I was on track to an above-average score for me. Then the next frame I bowled a strike, and the following frame I bowled another strike! At this point I did a little tapping before my next turn. There was pressure because I was going for the turkey on this one. I tapped on my fear of messing up the third strike and my fear of not getting a strike. I also tapped for five seconds or so after I picked up my ball. And sure enough, I got a third strike!

I was so excited, I yelled loud enough for everyone in the bowling alley to hear me. "I won a turkey!" My wife and kids all gave me high-fives. I ran over to the desk and had all the bowling alley employees give me a high-five. There were some friends of mine several lanes down, and I ran over to them and had them give me high-fives.

The next time I got the ball I tapped again, and I got another strike! Four in a row! And then I got another strike, and another one, and another one! Seven strikes in a row by the time the game ended. I bowled a 236, which is 100 points beyond what I thought would be a really good game. Our friends even asked me to come bowl on their lane so I could help them win a turkey. On their lane, I bowled another strike.

However, I started having some uncertainty because I didn't think the bowling alley wanted me to win a turkey for other people. Not surprisingly, the next frame ended the streak with a spare. I excused that by saying, "The ball slipped from my fingers," which it had, but I am almost certain it was because of those inner doubts about winning an extra turkey that I unconsciously "sabotaged" it.

The statistical probability of me bowling eight strikes in a row has to be near zero. EFT really works! It calms us down and removes doubt and fear, which in turn allows us to perform at the level we are capable of. Not only can it help with bowling, but every aspect of life —relationships, spirituality, money, professional goals, happiness, peace of mind, and the list could go on and on! EFT can help with so many things, it is awesome! Whenever it's appropriate, try EFT for yourself and others—miracles can happen!

※ ※ ※

If we are going to improve our performance at anything it is imperative that we remove our mental blocks to such achievement. That doesn't mean, however, that skill and practice are no longer necessary. Listen in as Judy Byrne in the U.K. uses these EFT principles to help an aspiring horse rider.

Becoming a Better Horse Rider

by Judy Byrne

"Jane" had very little riding experience as a child. When she was a young adult, she and a friend with even less experience went to a riding school and said they could both ride. The school believed them, gave them hard hats, put them on horses, and allowed them to go out into a field. After a while, Jane's horse got faster and faster. Then, when a nearby farmer began cutting his hedge, Jane's horse was spooked by the noise and went into a gallop, heading for a small stone wall. Jane thought she was going to die. But the horse stopped short of the wall and she fell off.

For a couple of decades Jane was frightened to be anywhere near horses. Now with cognitive therapy and a lot of guts she had resumed her confidence about being around a horse. She even offered to take care of one for someone else and had a few lessons on it. But she felt she was still "blocked." She said, "I cannot relax. My body stiffens. I am afraid when the horse goes fast, even when it is safe. My arms lock and become rigid. The horse feels this as a lack of support and he becomes anxious." She was really stuck in this cycle and felt frustrated.

We did the Movie Technique on her memory of the fall. As Jane processed it, she had some insights. What she had seen as the failure of falling off was actually something of a triumph for a novice rider to have stayed on as long as she did! She recognized that the trigger for her arms locking and becoming rigid now was the horse's head coming up, just as it had back then when she did not know how to stop it when it bolted.

When she could run the movie of the memory in her head with almost no distress, we changed to the Tell the Story Technique—getting her to tell me the story as if I had not heard it before and stopping to tap whenever any emotion came up. By the end of the session, she could tell the story without any emotion, we had tapped on a number of aspects that came up in the telling, and the memory had faded and become emotionally neutral.

But when she got home and reflected on it, Jane found her feelings about being on a fast horse fast had not changed. She said when I saw her a couple of weeks later, "I was so disappointed that I just cried and cried and cried. I had hoped for a Harry Potter magic wand. I did not have one."

Jane is not a woman who gives in easily. Despite her disappointment, the weekend after our session, she went for a lesson. As she got into it, she realized that her arms were no longer stiff. She was "open to the horse," comfortably taking in and responding to feedback from it. She was sitting better and riding better. She felt she was just "soaking the lesson up like a sponge."

Her teacher also noticed. She has a reputation as a great teacher but not one who uses praise for encouragement. She only acknowledges when people have really made progress. She confirmed Jane's perception that she was riding differently, and with promise of better yet to come.

Still, Jane was not quite convinced she had cracked it. She thought maybe the improvement would hold only when her teacher was there, telling her what to do. It was not until she had taken the horse out by herself and felt the same way that she started to be confident that she was now potentially quite a different rider.

When I saw her for the second and last time, I asked her to check out the original memory. It was like an old black and white photo and she realized she had hardly thought about it since the last session. Previously, it came into her mind often. An interesting sidelight on the way memory works was that Jane had stored it in her head as if she had seen it taken by a camera behind her. What she thought she remembered was quite different from anything she could possibly have seen.

And she realized that when you see a horse and rider that seem to "just flow together," it is because the rider is highly skilled and practiced. Top riders will ride up to six hours a day. There is talent but also a lot of craft in it. Once EFT had removed the block to learning, she still had to learn technique. The block had stopped her from seeing that before. Now that it had been cleared, the learning was only just beginning. She has to learn to be an expert rider. But I am betting nothing is going to stop her now.

❧ ❧ ❧

To some, this next report will be a trip into the ether. To others, it will provide evidence, and a possible EFT link, to the far reaching effects of our inner attitudes on our outer circumstances.

Almost everyone recognizes that we radiate our inner thoughts through such things as our posture, gestures, voice intonations, and choice of words. People pick up on this, of course, and tend to respond to us in a manner commensurate with what we are "putting out." Thus if we are internally angry, people will tend to be angry back. If we are internally peaceful, people will tend to give us peaceful feedback. Nothing new here.

But what about the effects of our internal state on the "non-people" elements of our outer world? Do our internal thoughts affect those as well? There have been many scientific experiments proving the effects of our intention on both living and inanimate objects. It is for real.

Along these lines Dr. Patricia Carrington provides us with the story of "Claude," whose ability to catch fish rose dramatically after using EFT to improve his inner states of embarrassment, jealousy, and lack of confidence. We can dismiss this account, of course, as being too "woo-woo"—or we can use it as evidence of exciting potentials within us. Which you choose, of course, depends on your inner thoughts.

Claude Improves His Fishing

by Patricia Carrington, Ph.D.

Speaking of using EFT "for everything" (Gary Craig's oft-repeated advice), I would like to report an unusual effect of this technique which was reported to me by Hank Krol, a counselor at Stairways Behavioral Health, an outpatient mental health clinic in Erie, Pennsylvania, which deals with severely disturbed patients.

Hank has developed a most interesting method of dealing with major depression using EFT. It involves breaking up the much-too-general category of "depression" into 15 component depressive symptoms, having the patient check those which apply to him or her, and then applying EFT to each one in turn, usually over a number of sessions. I will report here a rather puzzling effect of EFT experienced by one of the depressed patients Hank Krol has been treating.

"Claude" sought help at the clinic following a prolonged hospitalization for major depression. When commencing to treat him, Hank followed Gary's recommendation to demonstrate the efficacy of EFT right at the start when attempting to win newcomers over to the technique. He began by using EFT with Claude on relatively minor issues completely unrelated to his depression.

The first application was for a shoulder and lower back pain for which the tapping brought immediate relief. Claude's pain came down from an initial 7 or 8 on the 0-to-10 scale to a 1 by the end of the session, and Claude conceded that EFT was effective. When he returned for the next therapy session a week later, he had used EFT several times in the interim and in this way he had managed to keep his shoulder and neck pain minimal. He then asked Hank, quite out of the blue, if he thought EFT would "help me with my fishing."

Claude is semi-retired and one of his favorite pastimes is going down to the local creek where a number of experienced fishermen assemble daily. His girlfriend introduced him to fishing following his discharge from the hospital and he took to it right away. Being somewhat of a perfectionist, he bought all the right equipment (the very best) and carefully observed the other fishermen, making sure to use exactly what they did, fish in the same area, and so forth. While on the one hand he looked forward to his new hobby, it had so far been extremely frustrating for him.

There were usually at least ten other fisherman lined up on the bank and, according to Claude, almost all of them would manage to catch large numbers of big steelhead trout (Erie is a top city in the world for this variety of fish) each time they fished. By contrast, although the creek is known for its exceptional trout, Claude would consistently leave at the end of the day with only a couple of "small fish," if any, in his pail.

This was particularly frustrating because to his knowledge he was doing nothing differently from the other fishermen, but rather following their procedures "to the letter." He recalled that he fished with minimal luck on at least 15 to 20 different occasions and did not experience a single successful day during that time.

Claude was persistent, however, and he kept on fishing. In fact, he was wearing his fishing boots at this session and preparing to return to the creek right after his appointment.

Hank responded to Claude's question about using EFT for fishing by saying, "Let's try it." It is important to note, however, that Hank did not have Claude address his fishing problem as "the problem." That is, he did not suggest that he tap on "Even though I'm a failure at fishing…" or similar statements. Instead he questioned Claude about his *emotional* reactions to the failure and asked Claude to tap only on his feelings.

Claude was able to identify three primary emotional reactions to this situation—*jealousy, embarrassment, and a feeling of lack of confidence*—emotions that were quite familiar to him in other situations as well. When he tapped on *embarrassment,* his intensity was originally a 10 and after three rounds it had come down almost to zero. *Jealousy* was substantially reduced by the end of the session, and *lack of confidence* was similarly lessened. Claude was pleased with these results and marched out to test them at the creek.

When he returned for his next session he said, "I can't believe it, but that tapping worked for the fishing!" Here is his account of what happened.

When he went to the creek after his therapy session, the other fishermen were lined up and as usual were pulling in fish after fish. Claude set up his fishing gear and waited. But this time he didn't have to wait long. The fish began biting soon after he arrived there, and he found himself, to his amazement, bringing in so many steelhead trout that soon he had caught more than he could possibly use—and they were big ones, too!

This was the beginning of a new era. Claude systematically used EFT each day before he fished, and each time that he tapped away his embarrassment and jealousy and lack of confidence, he kept on having successes. He estimates that since he began using EFT, he has experienced 30 to 40 truly "good" fishing days and only 12 days that were "not so good," a remarkable record for him. At this writing, his success at fishing continues, contributing greatly to his self-esteem.

Asked how he explains his extreme lack of success before he learned EFT, Claude says that he attributed it to "bad luck" and that he had been "unlucky" all of his life. While he also lacked fishing experience, the fact that there was an immediate turnaround on the very day he commenced using EFT strongly suggests to him that "bad luck' really didn't have much to do with it. He says that when he taps on the three issues (embarrassment, jealousy, and lack of confidence) before he goes fishing, which he does religiously, he goes to the creek expecting to catch fish and that his lack of confidence is gone.

Although we can speculate on the reasons for the unexpected outcome, actually none of us know exactly how EFT worked to achieve its results from the standpoint of the fish. Since using EFT for this issue, is Claude now engaging in some uncharacteristic behavior when fishing that has turned the outcome around for him, even though he is not aware of behaving differently when using EFT? Obviously if he is doing this it is not apparent to him, and it is hard to imagine how confidence or lack of it is conveyed to the fish so that they either take the hook or not.

Those who have studied the operations of energy fields have observed that subtle energies are not confined to the individual but can impact many other organisms and sometimes even inanimate objects, as in the studies of the effects of thought on random number generators conducted by Robert Jahn, Dean of the School of Engineering at Princeton University. Reasoning from this perspective, one might wonder if Claude's much more relaxed and confident attitude about fishing is somehow being conveyed to the fish through means other than the five senses.

But all this is speculation. I leave it to you to decipher the mystery of the steelhead trouts' response to EFT.

❊ ❊ ❊

Rebecca Marina works out with weights and, of course, runs into "limits" regarding what her body will endure. She added EFT to her workout routine and was able to substantially improve her "reps." This is an important article because it points the way to performance enhancement of all kinds.

Using EFT for Weight Lifting

by Rebecca Marina

I have been lifting weights for a while and decided to add some EFT to my routine to see what would happen.

This morning I was doing "arms and upper body" and, it being Monday, I was feeling like I just wanted to hurry up and get it over with. I had already done sets of "pec flys," overhead presses, pull downs for the front and pull downs for the muscles in the back. So my muscles were feeling a bit tired.

I was just going into my third set of biceps and they were burning like fire (believe it or not, trainers consider this good), and I thought, *Why am I letting this be so hard when I have good ol' EFT to help me?*

So, just before my third set, I took a mini break to apply some EFT. I used the Setup Phrase:

Even though my arms are already burning like fire, I allow this set to be easy and free.

Sure enough, it worked like a charm! I could tell the difference especially because my arms were already fatigued and I usually barely get through my last set of biceps.

Next came shoulders. I always save shoulders for last because they hurt the most and I hate doing them. For this exercise, you stand up with a heavy weight in each hand and try to raise them outward, sort of like you are trying to fly. Well, it fatigues the muscle very quickly and it just downright hurts! So this time, I started out with a little EFT.

Even though I HATE doing shoulders, I choose to let them be light and free.

I then did my first set (I always do three sets of each exercise). It was much easier! On this particular exercise, I usually can only lift the weights up about eight times and I am just dying by the eighth one. This time I lifted it 12 times fairly easily! I did another round, also 12 times. By this time, EFT or no, my shoulders were quite fatigued and I still had one more set to go. So I stopped and did EFT saying,

Even though my shoulders are tired, I am asking extra blood and oxygen to flow to them and for this set to be easier than the first.

Well, It was! I easily went for 17 reps this time. I felt I had a really good workout. EFT can help you be the very best at anything.

I have used this same technique to help my son swim farther than he ever had. I don't know why I didn't think of using it right away on the weight lifting. Sometimes we get so busy tapping for everyone else, we forget about our own needs.

The weight lifting area is a virtually untapped market for EFT practitioners. Weight lifters will do almost anything to improve their performance. The money body builders and weightlifters spend on supplements will astound you! They can surely afford to spend some on an EFT practitioner who can help them attain, much more easily, the goals they are striving for.

I hope this encourages you all to apply EFT to your own workout routines.

❊ ❊ ❊

Here's a clever idea from Andi Whitaker of the United Kingdom. Andi shows how to enhance performance by tapping along with what's playing on the television set. Her approach might motivate even the most dedicated couch potato!

Tapping Along with the Olympics

by Andi Whitaker

Watching the Olympics on television, I have found it both inspiring and exhausting to see all that sweat and effort running across my TV screen every night.

Suddenly, after I had recovered from associating too strongly with a synchronized diving event, I had this brain wave. I could tap as I watched the finest athletes on the planet running across my lounge wall.

So I started tapping while saying:

Even though I cannot run fast enough, I deeply and completely accept myself. I could run faster. I could be more supple. I have a fantastic fit body. I can do press-ups easily.

I tapped so much my head started to fizz, a bit like recovering from a mild flu.

I continued this procedure over the remaining nights of the games and the results were very good. I have recently started a keep-fit program, involving four simple exercises and running in place. Before tapping in the manner indicated above, my best running in place achievement was 150 steps—and I was exhausted at the end of it. However, after tapping I easily reached 225 steps and five days later reached 400 steps. All this without straining. I was able to relax into the exercises in a manner that was previously impossible.

I have continued to maintain my progress and really enjoy the exercise program. Obviously the principle could be applied to any sport.

※ ※ ※

Marian Slaman from Toronto, Canada, found herself intimidated on a high-speed ski slope. So she used EFT while on the chair lift to help her stay relaxed and maintain control on the subsequent ski run. Each successive "EFT session on the chair lift" resulted in improved performance.

Mom Uses EFT to Improve Ski Performance

by Marian Slaman

When my son was seven, I dusted off my rusty ski legs and donned the slopes once again. Over the last few years, I have gone from teaching him how to ski to having to keep up with him on the slopes.

Last year I began skiing up the walls of the half pipe and taking in more jumps in the terrain park. In both cases I was somewhat (to put it mildly) intimidated by my environment, particularly in the half pipe where the speeds quickly increase. I am very conscious that in skiing, particularly at increasing speeds, it is important to stay relaxed and in the moment so that one can take the jumps and turns while staying connected to the snow, the hill, and ever-changing conditions as one proceeds down the hill. If one tenses up too much there is an increased chance of making a mistake and thus falling and injuring the body. Terrain park skiing is not for the faint of heart. As I came out of the half pipe and was aware of my fear, I realized that at my fingertips I had a solution.

I wanted to reduce my fear of going fast and reduce my tension level. I completed my run and on my next chair lift ride (in Ontario the runs are short) I tapped on issues related to staying in control, staying relaxed, and being comfortable with faster speeds.

On the next run down, I noticed an immediate improvement. With each successive run, I tapped a bit on the lift while ascending the hill and continued to reach increasing levels of comfort while descending. I was able to ski at increasing speeds while achieving tricks that are more complex with a feeling of comfort and control. With this I know that my skiing abilities can now improve at an increasing rate. Some of the Setup Phrases I used were:

Even though I get scared when I go fast, I deeply and completely accept myself.

Even though I am not use to skiing this fast.... Even though I haven't done this before.... Even though it is hard to go slow in the half pipe.... Even though I have never skied up walls before.... Even though I am not use to horizontal skiing.... Even though there isn't much room for slowing down.... Even though I haven't done jumps this high before.... Even though I feel as if I am too old for this.... Even though I feel I have to keep learning.... Even though I feel I have to keep pace with my son.... Even though I am afraid I will lose control, fall, and hurt myself....

I did two rounds of tapping, using as Reminder Phrases *lose control, lose control and fall,* and *hurt myself.*

I choose to ski relaxed. I choose to ski in control.

Even though my fears are taking me out of the present, I can stay in the moment

My 12-year-old son tasted snow boarding last year and has converted. He is now eager to trade in his skis for a snowboard. I promised him I would try out snow boarding when we go and a date has been set. I intend to bring along my EFT as I begin this new experience.

✿ ✿ ✿

Carol Tuttle is one of the most fit people you will meet and much of her fitness is due to her passion for running marathons. Carol started this demanding venture as a "marathon newbie" five years ago and, of course, had both physical challenges and limiting beliefs to overcome. She addressed both of these with EFT and gives all the details in this report.

How I Used EFT to Run 15 Marathons

by Carol Tuttle, Ph.D.

About 10 years ago if you had told me I was going to run a marathon—26.2 miles—I would not have believed you. The most I had ever run in my life was five miles and that had been over 25 years earlier. But deep within me there was a desire to collapse those limiting beliefs and take on the challenge. I knew that I would face many issues and blocks along the way so I decided to make EFT a part of my training and marathon running program.

Since time was an issue and I knew that I would be using more and more of my time each week to increase my miles, I incorporated my EFT "sessions" into my runs. A popular running program for newbies like me is a run/walk routine where you run for nine minutes and then walk for one minute. I used my one-minute walking time to do my EFT sessions.

Not only did I do this for all my runs for the eight months of training before my first marathon, but it worked so well that I used it for all the marathons I have run. Further, I will continue to use it.

I went through several stages during my training and many issues and limiting beliefs came up. I tapped using EFT's Basic Recipe while repeating the following Setup Phrases:

Even though I can't believe I am doing this, I am excited to take on the challenge.

Even though it scares me that I may die trying, I am letting go of the fear.

Even though I have never run that far for that long, I am going through all the steps that will prepare me to succeed at my goal.

As the miles began to increase week by week, I included statements like:

Even though I don't feel like getting up so early and running so far, I am staying true to my goal.

Even though I don't feel like running right now, I am committed to the outcome.

Even though I would rather stay in my bed, I am getting up now.

After tapping statements like those above I would continue tapping while repeating Reminder Phrases, tapping out all of the:

Fear / tired / why am I doing this / I am not a runner / what was I thinking / I don't know if I can do this...

After collapsing those negative thoughts and feelings I anchored in these positive beliefs by tapping and repeating:

I am proud of myself / I am ready to run / I am getting stronger and stronger each week / I am doing it even if it is hard at times / my body is strong and clear / I am grateful for my legs that they are willing to work this hard for me / I am achieving my goal and successfully running my first marathon.

Using EFT during the actual marathon run, I started by saying:

Even though I am not sure if I am ready for this, I am excited to be here with all these people who are here doing something great for themselves.

Even though I had to get up really, really early, I am rested and prepared.

Even though a lot of people are faster than me, I am grateful I am healthy enough to be doing this.

During my one-minute walking time, I use statements like:

Even though my legs are getting tired, I am strong and clear.

Even though this mile seems really long, I am pleasantly distracted and the time goes by quickly.

Even though I want to stop, I am choosing to keep on going and going.

Even though most people believe mile 20 is like "hitting a wall," I am fresh and just starting my run. The last 20 miles were just my warm-up!

I also include Reminder Phrases for tapping out all the:

Tiredness / burning / heavy / can't do this / what was I thinking / just want to stop / not sure if my body can keep on going / uncertainty…

I also made sure I tapped on positive statements to recharge my body with positive energy:

I am strong / I am clear / I am a great runner / I am experiencing the time going by quickly / I am nearly done / I am grateful for my strong healthy body / I am thankful for my legs / I am proud of my body and its willingness to do this.

I am here to tell you that using EFT in my training has made all the difference. Crossing the finish line of my first marathon was a spiritual high for me. Using EFT as part of my marathon training was so successful that I went on to run 15 more marathons in the next four and a half years. In 2005 I decided to switch from marathon running to competing in Sprint Distance Triathlons, and I have completed 17 triathlons to date. EFT helped me achieve my goal of competing in one triathlon a month from April to November in 2008, for a total of eight triathlons.

❉ ❉ ❉

EFT'ers report many interesting EFT "side effects" and this one by Masha Blaznik from Slovenia takes its rightful place among them. This may be quite useful for those who would like to feel motivated to exercise or even athletes who growl tired of training. Note how her main use of EFT centered around the Personal Peace Procedure, which is described at the end of Chapter One. Masha refers to EFT's fingertip tapping points, which are part of the full Basic Recipe described in Appendix A.

EFT for Exercise Motivation

by Masha Blaznik

I've been practicing EFT on myself, family, and friends for two years now. I'm excited and surprised in a positive way with the effect that this technique has on me personally. I've been trying it for everything and using the Personal Peace Procedure when stuff from the past came up. And the results are mindblowing!

I have never been keen on sports and loathed the faintest idea of working out. But I woke up one day with the need to exercise! I thought it would go away, so I waited. But the feeling that it would help me physically, mentally, and emotionally kept growing stronger. So I stared to jog. And it wasn't easy. Many memories and complexes came up that were related to sports and working out. I jogged while at the same time tapping on my finger points for a month.

After a month I stared to enjoy my runs and issues from the past were simply dissolved. Whenever I felt a physical symptom or emotional issue rise during my exercises, I tapped on my fingertips. In my experience, those fingertip tapping points are as effective as facial ones and I felt the results in seconds.

After three months of exercising, I ran the 10.5-kilometer (6.6-mile) marathon. And I was successful! I felt on top of the world! This technique has helped me to pursue the changes that I want in my life. I can feel and see them happening. It's amazing!

❅ ❅ ❅

Over the years we have received many reports about how people successfully used EFT by tapping on themselves on behalf of others. This is called surrogate EFT. You simply tap on yourself as though you are the other person. Surrogate tapping can be used to help pets and other animals as well as people of all ages, who can be in the same room with you or on the other side of the planet.

This surrogate tapping may seem quite strange—even laughable—to uninformed skeptics. However, the reports are far too numerous too ignore, and this report from Madelein Walker in South Africa is flat-out stunning. If you haven't tried surrogate EFT, this article should motivate you to do so.

Surrogate Tapping in a Large Cycling Race
by *Madelein Walker*

My friend Elsie and I are both newcomers to EFT and have loved it since the day we started. Our first experiment with surrogate tapping happened here in Johannesburg, South Africa, with a 78-kilometer (48-mile) cycling race. We agreed that I would not do any tapping at all but would phone her with all my aches and pains. She would then "tune in," as she calls it, and tap on herself for whatever I needed in that moment.

It worked brilliantly! The headache I had disappeared almost instantly and I finished the race in record time!

Then we really put it to the test. Elsie would do surrogate tapping for me when I rode the Argus, which is the biggest timed cycle race in the world with about 36,000 cyclists racing 108 kilometers (67 miles) over mountains and steep hills in our beautiful city of Cape Town!

Because she would be 1400 kilometers (870 miles) away and I wouldn't be able to use my cell phone while navigating through thousands of cyclists, we decided on a strategy. Elsie had a basic list of things that are always a problem for me during long cycle races, for which she would tap on the hour whether I phoned her or not. The list included painful quadriceps (from quick tiring and the wind chill factor), mental attitude (my self-talk turns negative when the going gets tough), energy levels (they fluctuate), and a runny nose (one of my big problems; it happens all the time). She would record what she tapped for and when.

My husband and I flew to Cape Town on the morning of 12 March 2005 for the race the next day. The Cape Southeaster Wind started blowing with all its might! The wind blew so fiercely, it sounded as if the windows were going to be ripped from their frames! We hardly slept that night and had to get up very early for our different starting times. My husband had a nice early start time but I started much later that morning. The later you start, the worse the wind factor.

I was so tired I couldn't keep my eyes open and was very tempted to do some tapping but decided not to in order to stay true to our experiment. I phoned Elsie while waiting to be loaded in my pen and asked her to tap for my tiredness, low energy levels, and pre-race anxiety. I didn't think about the wind as it was quiet within the city.

I specifically took my focus away from any expectations I had, sat down next to my bicycle, and just watched the people and their funny outfits. By the time my group was ready to go 15 minutes later, I realized that the tiredness was gone and I was calm and focused enough to tackle the race. I sent Elsie a cell phone text message to let her know she was spot on and that it was working. The gun went off, and there we went!

While cycling within the city on the way out, everything was fine and there was no sign of wind. But as soon as we headed onto the highway, the wind literally blew people all over the road and some went into a panic state. "Watch out!" "Keep your line!" The shouts echoed around me and I knew that I would either have to face my worst fear or return on a sweeping vehicle!

As negative thoughts flooded my mind, I felt myself getting more and more tired. All within the first hour of the race! I was setting myself up for failure!

By the time it was safe enough to stop, I realized I didn't need to! My legs were pumping and even though I had to hold on to my bike for dear life, I was doing just fine!

Unbelievable! I just kept going and going! I had to stop twice to adjust my helmet as it was almost blown off my head. I kept on going, and strangely, I started overtaking more and more people. Usually people overtake me!

Then I noticed that I hadn't once needed to blow my nose. My nose was as dry as a bone!

At about 63 kilometers (39 miles) to go, I stopped at a watering point and gave Elsie a quick call. The wind was so bad that I could not hear her on the other side, but I told her to continue to tap and do whatever she was doing because it worked magic!

Even when we were stopped at the top of Chapman's Peak for 25 minutes so they could airlift someone who had a heart attack, I remained positive and strong.

Of course the stop affected my overall time and the last 25 kilometers (15 miles) became stressful and dangerous. My nerves were shot going down the rest of Chapman's Peak at a very high speed amongst thousands of cyclists who had by now caught up. Suikerbossie, a very long and steep hill, became one big sea of people all trying to get to the top at the same time while still fighting the wind. But in spite of my nervousness, I remained strong and positive.

My husband couldn't believe his eyes when he saw me arriving back with a medal in my hand! He expected to see me in a sweeping vehicle because he knew how much I hated cycling in the wind, and I am generally not strong enough to keep up.

I phoned Elsie the first instant I could sit down and catch my breath. I was exhilarated and could almost not explain in words what effect her tapping had on my race. I know in my heart that if it wasn't for her and EFT, I wouldn't have finished the race!

Elsie had realized that the famous Southeaster was blowing after seeing it on TV about an hour into my race. She immediately started tapping with phrases like:

Even though the wind is strong, I am cycling strong and I positively accept myself. I feel comfortable and the wind doesn't bother me.

Even though the wind is causing discomfort in my body and my arms are sore from holding on so tightly, I deeply and completely accept myself.

Even though I have this fear of strong wind, I deeply and completely accept myself. I feel safe and I am having a safe ride.

Even though I am almost there, I am still motivated, I am still cycling strong and I have enough energy to finish the race.

I was ready to give up within the first hour of my race, and as soon as she started tapping, I had a change in cognition, motivation, and physical strength!

The other miracle was my running nose. She tapped once at the beginning of the race for that and I had a dry nose for the whole race! I went cycling again without tapping and my runny nose was back.

Surrogate tapping is so different from conventional EFT that it's easy to assume it can't make a difference, but my results were so unusual and spectacular that to me they are proof that EFT works — even if you are 1400 kilometers away from the person who is tapping on your behalf.

❦ ❦ ❦

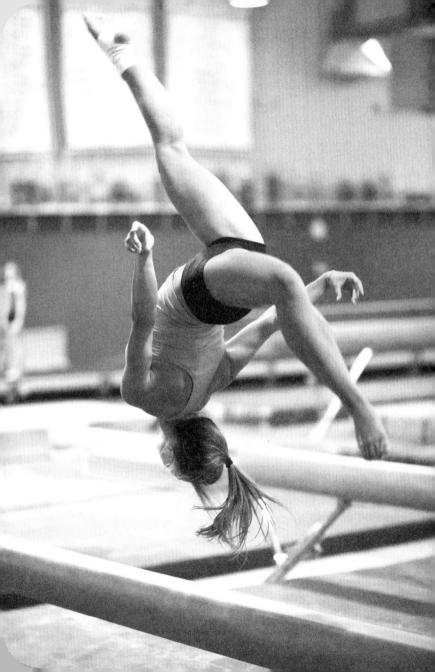

7

An EFT Success
Story In Detail

This next report is so comprehensive, it deserves its own chapter. Carol Look details for us a successful 90-minute session with a nationally ranked gymnast.

Sometimes a client thinks a problem that was successfully handled by EFT either "comes back" or that the work was "undone." Usually this is not the case, even though that is the client's clear perception.

Often, what "comes back" is simply another aspect of the same problem that was not uncovered in the original session. On other occasions the problem is actually a reaction to some substance to which the client is sensitive. In energy tapping terms, this has become known as an "energy toxin."

Carol illustrates this "energy toxin" phenomenon in her follow-up report.

Long-standing Fears
Fade for 19-year-old Gymnast

by Carol Look

Ann, a nationally ranked gymnast, had been struggling with an intense fear or phobia of back tumbling, which is a major part of her gymnastics routine. She was then 19 years old and had been competing in gymnastics since age eight. The executive coach hired by her parents to address the phobia referred her to me after hearing about my EFT work. In a single 90-minute session, the young gymnast recovered from her nine-year-long phobia.

While the following is not an exact transcript of my session with Ann, it accurately reflects the sequence, essence, descriptions, and details of our work together. I thought it would be helpful written in this format.

August 22, 2000

Carol: Your coach told me you have a lot of fear about your back tumbling routine. Tell me what happens to you and what it feels like.

Ann: I just got the shivers when you asked me that. That's how bad it is.

Carol: On a scale of zero to 10, where does it fit?

Ann: I would rate it a full 10 when I think about it now.

Carol: Even though you're not performing now?

Ann: Right. At least a 10. Way up there.

We started tapping:

Even though I'm afraid of back tumbling, I deeply and completely accept myself.

We tapped one round of the Basic Recipe.

Carol: Now check in and reevaluate the 10 you felt before.

Ann: It's definitely gone down to about an 8.

Carol: Good. Now tell me anything else that seems different about the fear when you imagine yourself doing your back tumbling.

Ann: OK. Now I'm standing at the tumbling strip, my coach is saying, "Let's go," and I can see myself lifting up my arms to start, returning them to my sides, pressing my hands down, and taking the deep breath I take before I begin.

Carol: What is all that?

Ann: That's what I do in preparation, my pre-tumbling moves.

Carol: This is different than before?

Ann: Yes, before I could only see myself standing there, feeling afraid. Oh, and now I can see some of my teammates around me.

Even though I'm still afraid of back tumbling and losing control…

Carol: Now tell me what's happened to the 8 and tell me if anything else has changed.

Ann: It definitely went down again. Maybe a 6 or so. OK, we're in season now, because I can see we're in a mock meet and all of my teammates are around me. My coach says, "Let's go," and I raise my arms, return them to my sides, take a deep breath, and then take my first step to do my back flips.

Carol: And what's significant about this scene?

Ann: I can actually see myself competing without being afraid. It also means I'm comfortable enough to be with my teammates. I'm usually too embarrassed when they see my fears.

For the next two rounds we tapped for:

Even though I dread doing back tumbling...and losing control...I deeply and completely accept myself.

Carol: Return to the same scene and tell me what you notice.

Ann: Now we're all standing in a circle with our hands in the middle because we're in competition! My coach says, 'Be great!" and I'm up first.

Carol: Is that unusual?

Ann: Yes, I never go first.

Carol: OK, then what?

Ann: I make my salute to the judge, and I complete my routine, and I'm really excited! I did it!

At first Ann's face looked totally different. She was beaming.

Then she started crying with relief. She said she hadn't felt this good since she was 10 years old. We did not rate any remaining fear. Clearly her distress had subsided.

I then asked her to tell me what happened when she was 10. She reported that her coach had been verbally abusive, demanding that she do 100 sit-ups whenever she felt afraid or hesitated at the back tumbling. She was able to talk about her coach without too much agitation until she linked the coach with her mother. Then she burst out crying and revealed how her mother had relentlessly pushed her, screamed at her, and punished her when she didn't complete her routines. She described how her mother would wait for her every day during practice, looking through a window into the gym. Ann said she never understood what she had done wrong when her mother would scream at her in the car. She held out her hand and said, "Look, I'm shaking just telling you about it." Her mother said phrases such as, "You're pathetic that you can't do better….You do the same @# %t# every day….You're not the only one who's going through this, you know…."

Even though I don't understand why my mother made me feel this way, I deeply and completely accept myself.

Even though I was afraid of her yelling at me…

Even though I felt helpless against my mother…

Even though the pitch of her voice was unbelievable…

Ann: Now I'm not looking at her. I get into the car, turn on the music, ride home with her and go upstairs to do my homework.

Carol: And tell me what's significant about that.

Ann: It never went that way, but it makes me feel in control, like I have a choice, and my stomach just released the way my shoulders released during the first round. My face feels better too. It usually gets really tight when I'm upset.

We tapped for several more rounds on incidents between Ann and her mother that still left her shaking. Again, she narrated new scenes and felt in control.

Ann: The new images give me power and control, what I've been so afraid of losing since I was 10. I think that's why I developed the phobia around that time.

Carol: OK. Now picture yourself in your gym back at college and tell me about anything that comes up that is disturbing or uncomfortable.

Ann: I don't see myself as very confident., maybe only a 4 out of a possible 10.

Even though I have terrible self-doubts about my gymnastic talent…

We continued to tap until she could picture herself confidently completing her routine in her gym.

Ann: Now I'm wearing my favorite leotard, my head is up, I see my coaches' pride, and the new freshmen say, "You look great." I'm at a 10 for confidence.

Ann had brought a five-minute videotape of her gymnastic routines that she used as a type of performance portfolio when applying to colleges. We viewed it four times in my office. I asked her to stop it anytime she felt a spike in her anxiety so we could tap for it. During the first viewing, she pointed out how her fear made her move too slowly in the forward tumbling and hesitate on the balance beam.

She tapped for her self-doubts and hesitation. The second time we viewed the tape, she tapped for her hesitation in the back tumbling. We tapped together until she said it looked like a past chapter in her life. She felt confident she no longer needed to tumble in a timid manner. While watching the tape for the third time, Ann tapped under her eye, her favorite spot, without using a Reminder Phrase, to clear out any remaining anxiety. The fourth and final time we watched the tape, she had me stop it when a friend landed off "the horse."

Ann: Look there, see how my friend landed? Recently, she blew out both her knees because of how she landed and I still have nightmares about it. I'm afraid I'm going to do the same thing.

Even though I'm afraid of blowing out my knees…

Even though I have this memory of my friend blowing out her knees…

We tapped until Ann could watch the whole tape without any feelings of discomfort or anxiety.

I didn't tell Ann that I no longer faint when I hear about someone's knee injuries, a problem that has apparently faded even though I have never tapped for it directly. I saw a friend high jump in sixth grade and "blow" her kneecap out. Unfortunately, I was still watching when the coach knocked her kneecap back in place. I've fainted three times in my adult life over "knee problems."

Ann practically did back flips when she left my office. She felt completely confident about returning to college and competing on her gymnastics team. She left her tape with me and I gave her my one-page quick reference guide for EFT. She was exhilarated and said she planned to tell her Olympic friends about the technique.

August 28, 2000

One week follow-up:

Ann called from college to ask a question about applying EFT to her doubts. She informed me she had her first practice that day.

Ann: I was awesome! Only one female coach was there. When I finished my routine, she was blown away. She couldn't stop talking about it. She said, "Who was that up there on the beam? You look like a new gymnast. What happened to you this summer? And where did you get all this confidence?"

Follow-up report:

After three weeks of excellent gymnastics practices, Ann called in a panic, telling me she had a "horrible" practice that day and had no idea what went wrong.

I asked Ann to describe what "horrible" meant to her. She said *"I wasn't myself"* and had pushed herself relentlessly to do a back tumbling routine instead of admitting that she was having a "bad day." She would not allow herself to back off and try again tomorrow. This was the first time since our session that she had felt any hesitation or fear. The experience spooked her, made her feel deeply fearful about future performances, and left her baffled as to why she would have had such a terrible practice. She also feared that all our work on her original phobic response had been "undone."

We explored what happened during the day that might have contributed to her fears. She said she had become intimidated after noticing an extremely talented freshman gymnast. She was unable to shake the feeling of intimidation and became determined to "compete" despite her better judgment. As a result, Ann didn't allow herself to back away from the tumbling mat when she should have, as she admitted all professional athletes need to do from time to time. She said she ignored her instinct to "call it a day" rather than push herself too far.

After we continued talking about her day, it seemed as if noticing the freshman gymnast was the only new emotional data that might have upset her and her energy system. However it still seemed unusual that she would have such a strong reaction and be unable to calm herself down from obsessive competitive thoughts and feelings of inadequacy.

Even though I'm intimidated by Cathy, I deeply and completely accept myself.

Even though I'm afraid I'm not good enough...

Even though I'm afraid of the competition...

Even though I'm afraid to be beaten...

Even though I need to be perfect all the time...

Even though I hate myself for hesitating...

Even though I'm ashamed of myself for not being perfect...

Even though I feel inadequate...

Throughout these rounds of Setups and tapping, Ann narrated her progress the way she had in our original session. She eventually landed in an emotional place of "feeling happy for Cathy" and "saw" herself cheering her on in the gym, unafraid of any rivalry. Ann said she now had a feeling that "there was enough to go around" and felt fully confident in her own abilities.

We talked about why seeing the freshman's performance had so unnerved her. She could not understand the strength of her reaction. It certainly was not the first time another superb gymnast had practiced with her.

Searching for an energy toxin, I asked, *"Have you eaten anything odd today, or used a new shampoo? Have you changed your perfume or were you wearing a new leotard?"*

Ann replied, *"That's funny you should ask. I accidentally put on my friend's cologne in the gym instead of my own and I couldn't get the smell off of me all day. It was awful."*

We had stumbled upon the culprit, a foreign scent that had disrupted Ann's energy system so deeply that once she felt intimidated, she could no longer soothe herself with any of her traditional resources, including her new tool of EFT. While the feelings of fear and intimidation were real and needed tapping, the energy toxin had reversed her in such a deep way that she couldn't correct her own energy system. In effect, she no longer had her wits about her and had admitted, "I didn't feel like myself."

We never actually tapped for the toxin itself. The tapping we did over the telephone left her feeling completely calm, reassured, and hopeful about her future performances. Ann no longer felt intimidated, scared, or self-hating. In fact, she had a hard time thinking about the freshman gymnast and decided that the whole experience was trivial rather than traumatic. And she was fascinated to learn about the power of energy toxins.

❖ ❖ ❖

Carol Look's report is worth studying for its many details. By asking meaningful questions and listening carefully, Carol was able to define the most important aspects of her client's problem, and incorporating Ann's own words into their Setup Phrases made the Setups more effective.

By having Ann imagine different situations in detail, Carol was able to test their results. She took this mental testing to a higher level by having Ann watch herself on video, and of course the final test took place when Ann went to her next practice. By tapping on every different aspect they could come up with, she and Ann successfully neutralized all of the memories and emotions that had interfered with her previous performance.

While *The EFT Manual* mentions energy toxins, I have found in recent years that they are usually less important than I had previously thought. Energy toxins include environmental factors like fluorescent lights, foods that the person might be sensitive or allergic to, and fragrances such as the one Ann encountered. Even though they're seldom a problem, when they are, they can really interfere with the process. If you're ever stuck or find that your EFT results seem to come undone, try tapping in a different room or outdoors or at a later time. A simple change in environment might produce a very different outcome.

✿ ✿ ✿

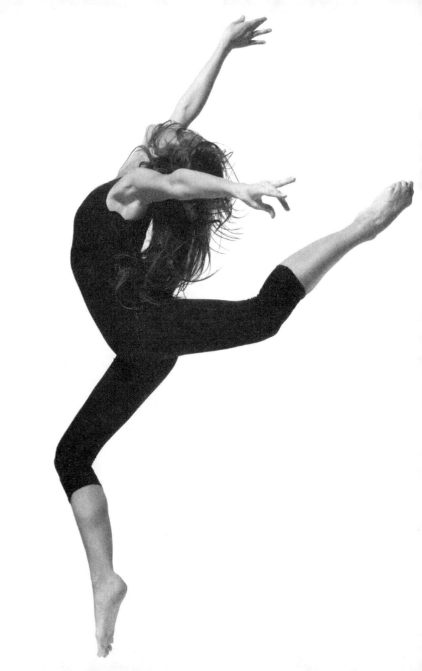

In Conclusion

Can EFT improve your athletic performance?

I believe it can, both in your favorite sport and in sports that are new to you or that so far haven't felt rewarding. It can even help you enjoy the training sessions and workouts that build strength, endurance, and coordination—exercises and activities that may not (yet) be on your list of favorites.

I would like to see EFT become an integral part of the preparation and training of athletes everywhere. EFT is truly a universal tool. It can be used by coaches, teams, and individual athletes. It can be used by people of all ages and all levels of skill and experience. It's hard to imagine a situation in which it can't make a positive difference.

That's because:

- The game that matters is the one in your head, and your greatest opponents are your own self-limiting beliefs.

- Your self-limiting beliefs didn't come out of nowhere —they came from past experiences and events.

- Tapping on the emotions that those past experiences and events still generate, thus reducing their power, is the fastest way to transform your self-talk at its source.

- Once self-limiting beliefs are neutralized, they can no longer interfere with performance or anything else, allowing you to relax and enjoy every aspect of your sport with significantly improved results.

As I mentioned at the beginning of this book, it's only natural for golfers to look for golf stories, for bowlers to look for bowling stories, and for baseball players to look for baseball stories. But the reports provided here are universal. They aren't sport-specific. The factors to look for are not the games or activities they describe but rather the emotional hurdles that their athletes overcame in order to improve or excel.

As you consider the changes or improvements you'd like to make, pay attention to your self-talk. Follow it back to the source, the events and experiences that created it in the first place.

Then focus on your feelings. Think about how you feel *now* about whatever happened *then*. Measure your anger, frustration, embarrassment, fear, or other emotions on the 0-to-10 scale. EFT stands for *Emotional* Freedom Techniques, and our target is always the *emotions*.

Try EFT's Basic Recipe as described in Chapter One. Most people experience at least some improvement from that simple formula.

As you review the different reports, think about how your own situation might be similar. Review the sections that describe aspects, core issues, the Movie and Story Techniques, the adjustment of your comfort zone, and tail-enders. These concepts are easy to grasp, and they are demonstrated throughout this book.

If you break a problem into its parts or aspects, if you focus on specific events, if you pay attention to the feelings and emotions those events generate, and if you tap on each aspect until you have neutralized its emotional charge, the problem will either cease to exist or become so insignificant that it no longer interferes with your performance.

The past ten years have brought EFT to a worldwide audience, and if you need help with your tapping, it's available through EFT training, in workshops taught by talented teachers, in one-on-one sessions with EFT practitioners, and in the many websites, books, e-books, videos, and other resources created by EFT specialists around the globe.

As interest in EFT's many sports applications grows, I hope that new books about EFT's use in individual sports will be published. My own contribution to this field is the e-book *EFT for Golf*. While it's true that EFT can be easily adapted to any sport, it's always interesting to see the many ways in which athletes, coaches, and EFT practitioners have applied it to a specific activity.

In the mean time, everything you need in order to start changing your life and your game is here in these pages. I wish you an exciting and rewarding journey!

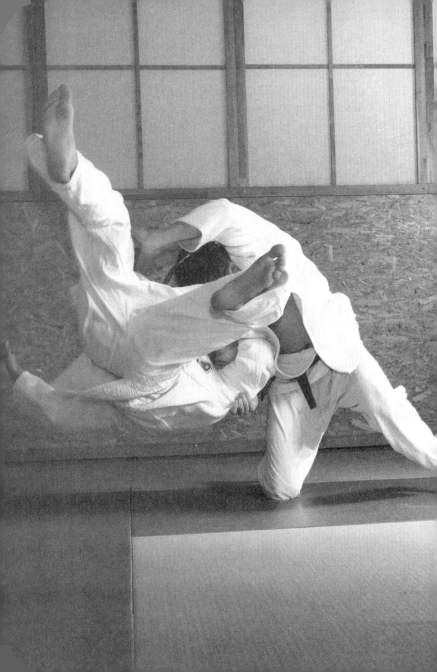

EFT Glossary

The following terms have specific meanings in EFT. They are often mentioned in EFT Insights e-newsletter, on the EFT website, and in *The EFT Manual*.

Aspects are "issues within issues," different facets or pieces of a problem that are related but separate. When new aspects appear, EFT can seem to stop working. In truth, the original EFT treatment continues to work while the new aspect triggers a new set of symptoms. In some cases, many of a problem's aspects require their own individual treatments. In others, only a few do.

Basic Recipe. The original EFT process is a four-step treatment consisting of Setup Phrase, Tapping Sequence, 9 Gamut Procedure, and Tapping Sequence again using EFT tapping points on the head, torso, and hands. The shortcut Basic Recipe, which is more commonly used, is a two-step treatment consisting of Setup Phrase and Sequence using EFT tapping points on the head and torso only. (See Chapter One.)

Borrowing Benefits. Tapping along with someone else's EFT session can provide surprising relief for your own issues as well. See also Easy EFT in Appendix B.

Core Issues. Core issues are deep, important underlying emotional imbalances, usually created in childhood or in response to traumatic events. A core issue is truly the crux of the problem, its root or heart. Core issues are not always obvious but careful detective work can often uncover them, and once discovered, they can be broken down into specific events and handled routinely with EFT.

Generalization Effect. When related issues are neutralized with EFT, they often take with them issues that are related in the person's mind. In this way, several issues can be resolved even though only one is directly treated.

Global. While the term "global" usually refers to something that is universal or experienced worldwide, in EFT it refers to problems, especially in Setup phrases, that are vague and not specific.

Intensity Meter. The 0-to-10 scale that measures pain, discomfort, anger, frustration, and every other physical or emotional symptom. Intensity can also be indicated with gestures, such as hands held close together (small discomfort) or wide apart (large discomfort).

Meridians. Invisible channels or pathways discovered thousands of years ago by Chinese physicians through which energy flows in the body. The basic premise of EFT is that the cause of every negative emotion and most physical symptoms is a block or disruption in the flow of energy along one or more of the meridians.

Movie Technique. In this process you review in your mind, as though it were a movie, a bothersome specific event. When intensity comes up, stop and tap on that intensity. When the intensity subsides, continue in your mind with the story. This method is commonly used by many EFT practitioners. For a full description, see www. EFTUniverse.com/tutorial/tutorcthree.htm

Personal Peace Procedure. An exercise in which you clear problems and release core issues one by one. Write down as many bothersome events from your life that you can remember (try for at least 50 or 100), then apply EFT to them one at at time until the emotional intensity fades. Eliminating at least one uncomfortable memory per day (a very conservative schedule) removes at least 90 unhappy events in three months. If you work through two or three per day, it's 180 or 270. See also Generalization Effect. For details, see www.EFTUniverse.com/tutorial/tutormthirteen.htm.

Proxy Tapping. See Surrogate EFT.

Reminder Phrase. A word, phrase, or sentence that helps the mind focus on the problem being treated. It is used in combination with meridian tapping points as a part of the Basic Recipe.

Setup Phrase. An opening statement said at the beginning of each EFT round, which defines and helps to neutralize the problem. In EFT, the standard Setup Phrase is, "Even though I have this _____, I deeply and completely accept myself."

Surrogate EFT. Tap on yourself as though you are the person or animal you wish to help.

Tail-enders. The "yes, but" statements that reflect negative self-talk. When you state a goal or affirmation, tail-enders point the way to core issues.

Tell the Story Technique. Narrate or tell the story out loud of a specific event dealing with trauma, grief, anger, etc., and stop to tap whenever the story becomes emotionally intense. Each of the stopping points represents another aspect of the issue that, on occasion, will take you to even deeper issues. This technique is identical to the Movie Technique except that in the Movie Technique, you simply watch past events unfold in your mind. In the Tell a Story Technique, you describe them out loud. For details, see http://www.EFTUniverse.com/tutorial/tutoritwelve.htm.

Appendix A:
The Full Basic Recipe

Although the shortcut version of EFT that's described throughout this book works well almost all of the time, the original version of EFT, which is described in *The EFT Manual*, contains additional features that are sometimes necessary. I recommend that everyone who's learning EFT become familiar with the full Basic Recipe, which includes tapping points on the fingers as well as the 9 Gamut Procedure. After you master the full Basic Recipe, feel free to put the finger points and the 9 Gamut Procedure on the shelf. As long as you obtain good results from the shortcut version, save time by using it—but if you feel stuck, try a few rounds of the original process.

Ingredient #1: The Setup

The full Basic Recipe begins with the Setup Phrase:

Even though I have this _____, I deeply and completely accept myself.

While reciting the Setup Phrase, either tap on the Karate Chop point or massage your Sore Spot.

The Sore Spot (described below) is not part of the shortcut EFT method described in this book, but it can be substituted for the Karate Chop point at the beginning of any EFT session. Here's how to find it.

The Sore Spot

There are two Sore Spots and it doesn't matter which one you use. They are located in the upper left and right portions of the chest.

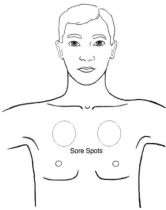

The Sore Spot.

Go to the base of the throat about where a man would knot his tie. Poke around in this area and you will find a U shaped notch at the top of your sternum (breastbone). From the top of that notch go down 2 or 3 inches toward your navel and sideways 2 or 3 inches to your left (or right). You should now be in the upper left (or right) portion of your chest. If you press vigorously in that area (within a 2-inch radius) you will find a spot that feels sore or tender. This happens because lymphatic congestion occurs there. When you rub it, you disperse that congestion. Fortunately, after a few episodes the congestion is all dispersed and the soreness goes away. Then you can rub it with no discomfort whatsoever.

I don't mean to overplay the soreness you may feel. You won't feel massive, intense pain by rubbing this Sore Spot. It is certainly bearable and should cause no undue discomfort. If it does, then lighten up your pressure a little.

Also, if you've had some kind of operation in that area of the chest or if there's any medical reason whatsoever why you shouldn't be probing around in that specific area then *switch to the other side.* Both sides are equally effective. In any case, if there is any doubt, consult your health practitioner before proceeding or simply tap the Karate Chop point instead.

Ingredient #2: The Sequence

The Sequence involves tapping on the Eyebrow, Side of Eye, Under Eye, Under Nose, Chin, Collarbone, Under Arm, and Below Nipple points.

The **Below Nipple** point is a newer addition to the full sequence. It was originally left out because it's in an awkward position for ladies while in social situations (restaurants, etc.) as well as in workshops. Even though the EFT results have been superb without it, I include it now for completeness. For men, it is one inch below the nipple. For ladies, it's where the under-skin of the breast meets the chest wall. Some call it the "underwire" point on an underwire bra. This point is abbreviated **BN** for **B**elow **N**ipple.

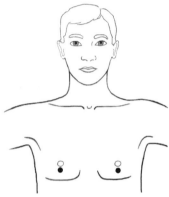

Below the Nipple (**BN**).

In addition, the Sequence in the full Basic Recipe includes the following finger points:

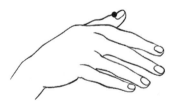

Thumb (**Th**) Point.

Thumb: On the outside edge of your thumb at a point even with the base of the thumbnail. This point is abbreviated **Th** for **Thumb**.

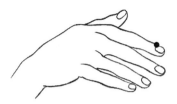

The Index Finger (**IF**) Point.

Index Finger: On the side of your index finger (the side facing your thumb) at a point even with the base of the fingernail. This point is abbreviated **IF** for **I**ndex **F**inger.

The Middle Finger (**MF**) Point.

Middle Finger: On the side of your middle finger (the side closest to your thumb) at a point even with the base of the fingernail. This point is abbreviated **MF** for **M**iddle **F**inger.

The Baby Finger (**BF**) Point.

Baby Finger: On the inside of your baby finger (the side closest to your thumb) at a point even with the base of the fingernail. This point is abbreviated **BF** for **B**aby **F**inger.

You may have noticed that the Sequence does not include the Ring Finger. However, some include it for convenience, and this does not interfere with EFT's effectiveness.

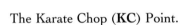

The Karate Chop (**KC**) Point.

Karate Chop: The last point is the Karate Chop point, which can also be used at the beginning of the Setup.

Thus, the complete Sequence consists of the following EFT points, which are tapped while one repeats a reminder phrase that describes the problem, such as "This headache" or "This fear of heights."

EB = Beginning of the **E**ye**B**row

SE = **S**ide of the **E**ye

UE = **U**nder the **E**ye

UN = **U**nder the **N**ose

Ch = **Ch**in

CB = Beginning of the **C**ollar**B**one

UA = **U**nder the **A**rm

BN = **B**elow the **N**ipple

Th = **Th**umb

IF = **I**ndex **F**inger

MF = **M**iddle **F**inger

BF = **B**aby **F**inger

KC = **K**arate **C**hop

Ingredient #3: The 9 Gamut Procedure

The 9 Gamut Procedure is perhaps the most bizarre looking process within EFT. Its purpose is to fine-tune the brain, which it does via some eye movements, humming, and counting. Through connecting nerves, certain parts of the brain are stimulated when the eyes are moved. Likewise, the right side of the brain (the creative side) is engaged when you hum a song and the left side (the digital side) is engaged when you count.

The 9 Gamut Procedure is a 10-second process in which nine "brain stimulating" actions are performed while one continuously taps on one of the body's energy points—the Gamut point. It has been found, after years of experience, that this routine can add efficiency to EFT and hasten your progress towards emotional freedom, especially when *sandwiched* between two trips through the Sequence.

One way to help memorize the Basic Recipe is to look at it as though it is a ham sandwich. The Setup is the preparation for the ham sandwich and the sandwich itself consists of two slices of bread (The Sequence) with the ham, or middle portion, as the 9 Gamut Procedure.

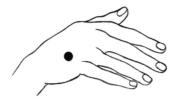

The Gamut Point.

To do the 9 Gamut Procedure, you must first locate the Gamut point. It is on the back of either hand and is 1/2 inch behind the midpoint between the knuckles at the base of the ring finger and the little finger.

If you draw an imaginary line between the knuckles at the base of the ring finger and little finger and consider that line to be the base of an equilateral triangle whose other sides converge to a point (apex) in the direction of the wrist, then the Gamut point would be located at the apex of the triangle. With the index finger of your tapping hand, feel for a small indentation on the back of your tapped hand near the base of the little finger and ring finger. There is just enough room there to tap with the tips of your index and middle fingers.

Next, you must perform nine different steps while tapping the Gamut point continuously. These 9 Gamut steps are:

1. Eyes closed.
2. Eyes open.

3. Eyes down hard right while holding the head steady.

4. Eyes down hard left while holding the head steady.

5. Roll the eyes in a circle as though your nose is at the center of a clock and you are trying to see all the numbers in order.

6. Roll the eyes in a circle in the reverse direction.

7. Hum two seconds of a song (I usually suggest "Happy Birthday").

8. Count rapidly from 1 to 5.

9. Hum two seconds of a song again.

Note that these nine actions are presented in a certain order and I suggest that you memorize them in the order given. However, you can mix the order up if you wish so long as you do all nine of them *and* you perform the last three together as a unit. That is, you hum for two seconds, then count, then hum the song again, in that order. Years of experience have proven this to be important.

Also, note that for some people humming "Happy Birthday" causes resistance because it brings up memories of unhappy birthdays. In this case, you can either use EFT on those unhappy memories and resolve them or you can side-step this issue for now by substituting some other song.

Ingredient #4: The Sequence (again)

The fourth and last ingredient in the Basic Recipe is another trip through The Sequence, including the finger points.

As in the shortcut Basic Recipe, check for any remaining discomfort, in which case you'll do another round of EFT tapping using a modified Setup Phrase:

> *Even though I still have some of this _____, I deeply and completely accept myself.*

You will add "remaining" to the Reminder Phrases as you tap through the complete Sequence.

Appendix B:
Easy EFT

Now I would like to introduce you to a fast, effective, and effortless way to learn EFT. It's literally as easy as watching a video and tapping along with it. You can use one of the many EFT videos at www.EFTUniverse.com for this purpose.

The Easy EFT technique may be the most important advancement in the healing field since EFT was first introduced. It puts the essence of this powerful process within easy reach of everyone.

Here are its three simple steps.

1. Identify the issues.

Write down a list of your issues, or the things you would like to improve, and rank their current intensities on a scale of 0-to-10. For example:

Neck pain: 7   Anxiety: 5   Emotional Overeating: 9

You can also tap for specific things that bother you, such as:

Angry at the clerk who was rude to me yesterday: 8

Upset about my son's accident last week: 7

Disappointed with myself for gaining five pounds this month: 9

Really hurt by my friend's criticism: 10

2. Tap along.

Fast-forward the video until you come to a tapping session. Then simply tap along as though you were the client on the screen. It doesn't matter which sessions you choose or whether they address your issues directly. Your system will empathize with the story and automatically target your issues behind the scenes.

3. Check your results.

Revisit your list of issues and write down their new 0-to-10 intensities. You should notice some improvement each time. The more sessions you tap along with, the better your results.

That's it!

But for best results, review the *Questions and Answers* and *Helpful Tips* below.

Questions and Answers about Easy EFT

Q: How was Easy EFT discovered?

A: I first discovered this process after EFT practitioners repeatedly told me that their personal issues improved as a result of tapping along with their clients. The first example occurred when I learned that someone's thyroid function improved. Next I learned that a fear of driving over bridges vanished. And then I got a barrage of reports regarding major improvements in fears, anxieties, anger, and trauma as well as a long list of physical symptoms.

But what's astonishing about this is that the EFT practitioners weren't tapping for their own issues—they were tapping along with their clients for seemingly different issues. This is a stunning discovery and means that our systems have the intelligence to "borrow benefits" and draw parallels from someone else's session. I find this happens with great regularity and, with Easy EFT, the same thing can happen for you.

Q: Why does Easy EFT work so well?

A: As you tap along with the authentic people featured on our videos, your system finds similarities between your issues and the ones being addressed on stage, *and you don't even have to know what they are!* This often happens in the background and allows the impressive meridian-balancing feature of EFT to go to work. It's a delight to use because it automatically injects the principles of EFT into something everyone enjoys doing …watching television.

Q: Can I really benefit from a session that deals with someone else's issue?

A: Yes! It's done all the time. If a housewife, for example, taps along with a session involving a war veteran's grief, fear, guilt, anger, and trauma, her system will bring up *her own* experiences of the same emotions. Tuning into someone else's issues this way is a natural thing to do and is commonly known as empathy. Easy EFT can then address these emotions and whatever physical symptoms might be associated with them.

Sometimes you might be aware that these issues are surfacing and you may feel some discomfort. Other times, things are being addressed in the background, outside of your awareness. How will you know if you are making progress? By assessing the 0-to-10 intensities as you persistently use Easy EFT.

Q: What should I expect?

A: Properly done, many of your results should range from "clearly improved" to "completely resolved." I cannot tell you in advance which of your issues will show the most improvement, but I can say that the more sessions you tap along with, the better your results can be over time.

Many people report much less emotional baggage and the reduction (or elimination) of severe physical symptoms, such as pain, allergies, addictive cravings, and so on. While I would expect that consistency will bring you great rewards, this does not mean that every issue will be resolved or improved.

Obviously, you cannot expect Easy EFT to be as thorough as OFFICIAL EFT. Some results may come right away, while others may take a while. Accordingly, anytime you want faster results, you can visit our website for a Certified EFT Practitioner, or learn OFFICIAL EFT yourself. Otherwise, persistence and patience will often pay off in a big way.

For perspective, I conducted this process one afternoon in Chicago for an audience of 500 people and 499 reported impressive results. However, this does not represent a guarantee. Your results may vary from this and there's a small possibility that you may not experience any benefits at all.

Q: Are there any cautions regarding this process?

A: While Easy EFT is relatively gentle and most people fly right through it with ease, it is possible that you may open up some stressful issues. Further, about 3 or 4 percent of the population (my estimate) have such frail emotional or physical issues that they should not attempt any healing aid on their own. Such attempts could lead to stress and unwanted results. Accordingly, you are advised to consult a qualified health professional before proceeding with this method.

Helpful Tips for Getting the Most Out of Easy EFT

Watch the EFT sessions on the web. This will acquaint you with the basic tapping points and make it easier for you to tap along.

- You do not have to read *The EFT Manual* to benefit from Easy EFT.

- You may find that the EFT sessions vary the method a bit and add new tapping points from time to time. These variations represent sophistications within EFT that are not necessary for you to understand for now. Any benefits they may provide will be automatically integrated within your Easy EFT results. Just tap along.

- **At first, you may find the tapping pace in the sessions to be too fast for you to follow along.** That's OK, just do your best. The process can still help you even if you miss a tapping point here or there. Eventually, you will get used to the process and the pace will be easy to follow.

Spend quality time with your list of issues and their 0-to-10 intensities because they are the foundation of this process. Don't just throw down two or three issues and guess at their 0-to-10 ratings.

- For your list, go back to childhood and pick up every anger, guilt, fear, etc. issue you can recall. Run through them mentally to see what **current** 0-to-10 intensities they bring up, not the way you felt when it happened. Then take an inventory of your body and list every pain or other physical symptom or disease you can find. List everything and don't skip something just because you think it is too big or "impossible."

- If you can't find a 0-to-10 intensity, that's OK. Just estimate what the number should be. It's amazing how accurate such estimates tend to be. The mere fact that you remembered an issue means you have some sort of charge on it, albeit possibly repressed. These can be helped by Easy EFT.

- List as many issues as you want. The more, the merrier. Fifty is better than ten because this gives Easy

EFT a wider doorway through which it can provide benefits.

- Your list might look something like the chart below after a few tap-along sessions. This example is for illustration only and does not indicate what you should expect on the specific items listed. Note that some of your issues will do better than others and some may not make much progress. **You will need to look at the overall picture to properly evaluate how well Easy EFT is doing for you.**

Issue	Original 0-to-10	Session 1 0-to-10	Session 2 0-to-10	Session 3 0-to-10	Etc.
Fear of Heights	8	5	2	3	
Easily Angered	10	10	5	2	
Test Anxiety	7	7	5	7	
Knee Pain	9	2	0	0	
Digestion Problems	4	4	2	3	
Etc.					
Etc.					
Etc.					

To find the tapping sessions, browse the free videos on the www.EFTUniverse.com until you find two or more people tapping together. Then rewind back to the beginning of the session and tap along as though you were the person being helped. It doesn't matter that your issues may be different from the people on stage. You will find that their issues will bring up yours. At the core, our issues are all very similar.

Some of your results may be subtle and you may not notice them until later. Further, you may also have some pleasant "side benefits" wherein improvements occur that you weren't expecting. Here are some examples:

Uncle Joe's aggressive personality may no longer bother you.

People may say that you seem more relaxed.

Your golf game may improve.

You may sleep better.

You may enjoy your work more.

Certain memories may no longer bother you.

Physical symptoms may improve.

Read your list of issues before each tap-along session just to remind your system of what you are working on. After that, put the list aside and ignore your issues —there is no need to keep focusing on them. Leave them alone so your system can draw on its wisdom and work on your issues in the background. Just tap along and enjoy the session while Easy EFT goes to work.

Revisit your list after each tap-along session. Then go through each issue and carefully assess any changes in current intensity. Write them all down, even those that haven't changed. Then do another tap-along session and visit the list again.

Do your sessions on any schedule you like. You can do them daily, weekly, or at any time interval you choose. You can even do several per day or break them up so that you do a half session today and finish it tomorrow. It all depends on your schedule.

Get plenty of EFT sessions to work with. There are books and videos at www.EFTUniverse.com that contain one or more sessions. In combination, they offer an impressive variety of issues from which to choose, and represent a lifetime of healing possibilities for you and your family.

Most Importantly…have fun with it!

EFT doesn't have to be complicated, difficult, or totally serious. You'll find plenty to laugh about in our EFT books, any EFT workshops you may attend, and your own EFT sessions at home.

EFT Resources

For information about EFT, including a free down-loadable Get Started package, go to www.EFTUniverse.com. On this web site, you'll find thousands of case histories of people who've used EFT successfully for every conceivable problem. You'll also find practitioner listings, tutorials, books, DVDs, classes, volunteer opportunities, and other resources to allow you to get the most from EFT.

My e-book supplement *EFT for Golf*, which describes how to tap for this sport in detail, is available from www.EFTUniverse.com and www.Amazon.com.

Index

A world of wellness at your fingertips!

To see more books in this series of authorized EFT guides, including....

The EFT Manual
EFT for Weight Loss
EFT for Fibromyalgia and Chronic Fatigue
EFT for the Highly Sensitive Temperament
EFT for Golf
EFT for Love Relationships
EFT for Abundance
EFT for Post Traumatic Stress Syndrome
EFT for Procrastination
EFT for Back Pain

Go to www.EFTBookShelf.com